# Natural Remedies For

# Cats

## Mark Gilberd

**Homoeopath. Medical Herbalist and Iridologist**

Text Copyright 2012 Mark Gilberd
Global Warming Edition 2024

# Index

# Welcome To the Animal Natural Remedy Series

These books are a effort to preserve the documentation of Natural Remedies used in the treatment of animals. In the past 100 years most of these treatments have been lost, especially in the treatment of cattle one of our most ancient of farm animals. Other reasons for writing these books is that I hate vet bills and people having to kill their farm animals or pets for economic reasons which I myself have been forced to do in the past on a Goat farm. Originally these books were put together as a field reference for myself for there is nothing worse than being in a paddock with a sick animal with the farmer, his hands on his hips waiting for you to perform and fix his animal.

Now the books have evolved and have had about 15 years of additions and are offered to you to teach you a new way of thinking. The books have evolved more by my different trainings. As a farmer I learnt to supplement the animals with the deficiencies of the soil so the books always start with the vitamins and minerals and their deficiency symptoms. As a Iridologist I tend to think and work with Body Systems such as The Nervous System or The Digestive System and concentrate on building them up with Nutrition and Herbs. As a Medical Herbalist I am trained to think holistically and design formulas that cover the whole being along with making the formulas easily absorbed. My Homoeopathic training teaches me to pay attention to the mind symptoms and to pay attention to what is really there not what I think is there and to treat and relieve the symptoms of the individual. Homoeopathy also shows how disease taints can be inherited and what to look for and how to treat them but best of all it gives me a special weapon to use when disaster strikes in the form of epidemics, these are called Disease Nosodes which are a preparation made from the disease product so you have a tool to help prevent the spread of disease. The books are set out in such a way as to teach you the correct use of Herbs eg thinking in body systems such as the Respiratory System or the Nervous System and in using herbs by their Medical Actions rather then that herb worked well last time. At the end of each system for example The Nervous System we have a section that gives you the common Actions used and needed for that section. Keeping with our example The Nervous System some of our

Actions would be Anti-spasmodic, Sedative and Nervine Stimulants. After the explanation of the Action you have a list of herbs that are known to be strong in that action, this gives you more of a selection of herbs then what is mentioned in the text. Next we move on to the Homoeopathic Remedies for the condition which have the details to allow you to select a reasonably similar remedy. Homeopathy sits on a three legged stool. What this means is that if a remedy has at least three symptoms in the same strength as the symptoms you are trying to match then that remedy is a potential cure for your patient or if not cure it will offer the condition relief. The more symptoms you can match to the remedy the better the remedy will work for the rule is likes cure likes not vaguely similar cures. Homoeopathy (homo means same pathy means disease) is a good form of treatment for animals who usually respond to it fairly well and also it is very cheap to use and very easy to medicate unlike the herbs. A lot of effort has been put into the symptom details of the disease as it is very hard trying to diagnose when the animal can't answer your questions, so here you have to be very observant.

If used correctly this book makes you think and act more like a Professional Herbalist and broadens your view on what you are doing. With the Homoeopathics I have only really given you the leading remedies to put you on the right track, it would be worthwhile to invest in a good Materia Medica (Homoeopathic Remedy Reference) such as Boericke's which is one of the best for the Layman.

## Main Reference Sources

The original base of the herbs I use were sourced from Juliette de Baïracli Levy's old Herbals, as hers are about the only Animal Herb References that have not been lost in time and they give you a lot of the old ancient herbs that have been used throughout most of history. To these I have added a lot of the more modern Herbs especially those that I use in my own work such as Astragalus and those that will soon be added after using for the first time on animals because there are just no substitutes. A good and recent example is Brahmi which I used in a cat recovering from a stroke because of my previous success in humans with this herb as it is supposed to rewire the brain around the damaged area and in its 3000 years of constant use someone must of used it on an Animal before. There are new herbs coming mainly from the Philippines, Indonesia, India and China but they are still being tried and tested and the average person wouldn't be able to get hold of them but the future looks far brighter than what it was 15 years ago when I started slowly putting this all together. We owe a lot to Juliette de Baïracli Levy for without her all these valuable herbs and how they were used would be lost. She has created a strong foundation that we can now build on.

**Juliette de Baïracli Levy (11 November 1912 – 28 May 2009)** was an English herbalist and author noted for her pioneering work in holistic veterinary medicine. Born to a wealthy Jewish family (her father was Turkish, her mother Egyptian) and raised in England with chauffeurs, maids, cooks, and gardeners. She knew as a child that she wanted to be a veterinarian. After studying veterinary medicine at the Universities of Manchester and Liverpool for two years she left England to study herbal medicine in Europe, Turkey, North Africa, Israel and Greece, living with gypsies, farmers and livestock breeders and recording their knowledge, especially the Gypsies. "I realized that if I wanted to learn the traditional ways of healing and caring for animals, I had to be where people still lived close to the land and close to their flocks," she says. "From Berbers, Bedouins, nomads, peasants, and gypsies in England, Israel, Greece, Turkey, Mexico, and Austria, I learned herbal knowledge and the simple laws of health and happiness. I never tired of traveling with my Afghan Hounds, always living with and learning from those around me." After living for some time on the Greek island Kythira she then resided in an old age home in Burgdorf, Switzerland leaving the world a better place.

For Homoeopathy my main hero is George Macleod not only for the success had based on his work but in my opinion he is a Homoeopathic Master up there with the greats and I admire his work in the use of Homoeopathic Disease Nosodes. All the high potencies mentioned are his work along with most of the Nosodes for as any trained Homoeopath knows and has had beaten into them during training you don't change the work of the masters.

Unfortunately in our fast paced world not many people have time for Homoeopathy but I will say this, in the next Global Pandemic I and my family will be safe because I will make the Disease Nosode of it for I was trained by the Homoeopathic Masters.

**George MacLeod (McLeod) (1912 – 1995) MRCVS DVSM Veterinary FF. Hom** was a homeopathic vet, President of The British Association of Homeopathic Vets, Veterinary Consultant to The Homeopathic Development Foundation. George MacLeod was a graduate of Glasgow University and was one of the world's foremost authorities on Homeopathic treatment of animals. He was one of the few veterinary surgeons to use Homeopathic medicines wholly and exclusively. He was responsible for keeping Homeopathy available for animals in the UK, almost single-handedly, for the middle part of the 20th Century.

Other animal Homoeopaths sourced are Christopher Day, Edward Ruddock, and John Rush

# Animal Natural Remedy Books

Natural Remedies for Cats
Natural Remedies for Dogs
Natural Remedies for Goats
Natural Remedies for Sheep
Natural Remedies for Pigs
Natural Remedies for Cows
Natural Remedies for Horses
Natural Remedies for Poultry

**Mark Gilberd, Homoeopath, Iridologist, Medical Herbalist**

# De-Sexing Your Animals

In Australia over 300,000 unwanted, homeless and abandoned cats and dogs are put down each year so why do we want to bring more in the world when we can't even look after what is here already. I believe it is best to wait till the animal is mature and its organs are fully developed before de-sexing. De-sexing is best done just after puberty for females maybe 6 to 8 months and for males you should wait a little while longer as they are more slow to mature then females maybe about 9 to 12 months. For males this is very important for later in life there is a big chance that they will suffer from urinary gravel or stones so you want the main pipe lines in the male to grow to maximum size before you de-sex them as doing it earlier could inhibit the growth in this area.

Animals that are not De-sexed may have mating urges that can lead to behaviour that is considered undesirable by some humans such as running away, fighting other animals of the same sex and getting injured, territorial marking, yowling and climbing walls, females being pursued by male animals, hyperactivity or aggression.

De-sexing does not take away the animals zest for life or make them lazy, it makes animals less prone to prostate cancer and reproductive diseases and on average they live longer.

# Vaccinations

I am very unsure about vaccinations and after reading of the side effects in humans from the manuals that Doctors use to vaccinate I find the whole idea fairly disturbing and I have never yet seen a document proving beyond a doubt that vaccinations truly work and there is just so much disinformation out there I don't think the truth will ever be known until it is possibly too late. It seems strange that Allopathic Medicine which usually always insists that they have to have proof, that there has to be double blind studies etc. and as yet we have never really seen the proof.     I know that animals suffer a lot of complications from the vaccines that they are given but when vaccinations make up a big part of your vets income and make the drug companies millions we will no doubt have to put up with lots more disinformation for many years to come.

I would be very interested in the results of a survey of how many vets vaccinate their own animals. A lot of you may be forced to vaccinate your pet if you ever put them in a veterinary hospital or ever need to board your cat or dog in a boarding kennel. The question to ask here if this happens to you is why should I vaccinate my animal when all of yours are already vaccinated or don't your vaccines work ?. I can see the argument they will use against this but let's use their claims against them, surely your animals should be safe because they have been vaccinated and obviously they can't give the disease to my pet because they have been vaccinated and can't get the disease.

The real truth I think is that vaccination is a numbers game, It only really works when most of the population is Vaccinated.

## If You Must Vaccinate

1.  Wait at least till the animal is 3 months old so the immune system has had a chance to mature.

2.  Never vaccinate a animal with symptoms of acute or chronic health problems, or at the time of surgery or any other physical or emotional stress.

3.  Try to vaccinate for one disease at a time allowing time for recovery and only use killed vaccines not live modified virus vaccines.

4.  Does a animal in good health on a good diet instead of the usual junk food diet really need boosters ?, and if you decide yes then why not do it every two to three years especially if your pet is in the middle years.

## Bad Effects of Vaccination

Signs of a negative vaccine effect are - erratic behaviour problems soon after shots, small warts, cancer, kidney failure, tumours, bloat of the stomach, skin problems, some say that 90% of skin problems are related to toxic vaccination and some animals have actually contracted the disease they were vaccinated for especially in Feline Leukemia and Parvo.

## Homoeopathic Treatment

If you suspect the cats or dogs illness is related to vaccinations directly after the vaccinations or three months down the track you can reduce the toxic side effects by using

**Thuja 30C** - as soon as possible dose nightly for seven nights then dose with **Sulphur 30C** weekly for seven more doses.

## Herbal Treatment

A natural antidote which acts as a body cleanser and as a detoxifier for vaccinosis reaction whether they are tumours or skin problems are a combination of **Sweet Violets** and **Red Clover.**

# Diet and Nutrition

## Our Supermarket Pet food

The supermarket and Pet Food manufactures do not provide safe food for our pets even though the adds tell us that they do but the simple fact is just read the can where it says Not Fit For Human Consumptio . If you can't eat it why expect your pet to. Now let's have a look where all this food comes from. 40% of the food comes from the rubbish parts of the slaughter trade being mainly feet, organs, blood, hides, hooves, beaks etc, (I know as I used to drive the tilt forklift with the buckets of offal which I used to tilt over the freezer while another person sorted by putting the heart in one section, liver in another etc) and we won't mention the animals that are diseased and cancerous that failed to meet the grade for human consumption. The remaining percentage of our supermarket pet foods consist of vegetable fiber, grain and chemicals. Vegetable fiber is made up of corn husks, peanut hulls, ground up corn and what a nutritionless waste it is. In many cases it is grain or soy meal which has been condemned from human consumption because of mold, debris, odors or bacterial contamination.

Next come the chemicals, but before we get to that lets have a look at the chemicals which are feed and medicated to the beef and poultry and other farm animal so as to bring them to slaughter earlier and allow them to live in crowded conditions, these mainly are hormones, steroids and antibiotics. Obviously these chemicals would be concentrated in some organs especially the liver which has the job of getting rid of them so they would be bound to pass on to all who eat them. Now add to these chemicals all the ones that are now added to preserve the product with the worst being Ethoxyquin (Find out about this one yourself especially who invented it and for what purpose as I don't want to be run over by a pet food truck). Now after this comes the artificial colouring, sugar (diabetes) and salt (blood pressure, kidney problems) which prevent the fat in the food from going rancid. Sugar can comprise as much as 25% of the semi moist dog food packets and dog biscuits. Sugar and salt can become addictive, resulting in diabetes, arthritis, cataracts, allergies, overweight, tooth decay and nervousness. In other words we have given them all our human problems which we get from eating processed foods. So next time you are in the supermarket buying pet food read the labels very carefully and ask lots of questions.

Let's have a look now what a proper diet should be.

## What the Diet Should Be

Dogs and cats are both carnivores which are flesh eaters and as such require a diet of flesh derived protein, raw meat is the central ingredient in a optimal diet. This meat for our pets should be of human consumption quality, fed raw because cooking destroys the vitamins, minerals and enzymes needed for digestion. Cooked and canned food is dead food for our pets and causes mucous to form in the animals intestines, mucous being the main food for worms and parasites.

A good diet would be of about 75% raw meat e.g. beef, poultry, fish etc. and about 25% vegetables. The Vegetables could include very finely chopped carrots, broccoli, sprouts, parsley, asparagus, garlic, sweet potatoes, squash, cauliflower, turnips etc.

The best type of food you can feed your cat or dog is the one you make yourself. It is the most natural, the most nutritionally balanced, the most easily digested and of much higher quality then canned or dry pet food.

Homemade pet food is not only free of harmful additives but has the added benefit of being able to include herbs. Two good ones that should be used frequently are garlic which is a natural anti biotic which has a high sulphur content which acts as a natural flea repellent (worms don't like it either) and the other herb is parsley that acts on the urinary system keeping it free from problems. A good diet produces a good and healthy digestive system which makes it very hard for worms and parasites to survive and also eliminates constipation. For those who feel that they do not have the time to prepare homemade food you will be happy to know that you can prepare it all at once and freeze maybe a week's worth at a time. Really it does not cost much more than what you spend on pet food anyway and just imagine how much money you will save yourself in future vet bills.

Let's take a look now at the digestive systems of cats and dogs and see why this diet is suitable. Cats and dogs do not chew their food for their teeth are for ripping and tearing and they swallow their food in chunks. Their digestive systems are much more acidic then ours and the small intestines are much shorter so meat goes through very quickly. Raw vegetables must be processed into very fine tiny pieces in order for the carnivore to digest them properly and be able to utilize them. In nature carnivores would get pre-digested vegetation while eating the stomach of a herbivore that they had killed. In preparing foods for our animals we do not have the option of feeding pre-digested vegetables so we must do what we can to provide raw ground vegetables which are as close to what mother nature would do as possible.

## The Cat Diet - Natural and Home Prepared

**60% Raw Meat** - Chopped or diced mutton, goat, roo, fish, organic chicken. (minced meat destroys vitamins). Once a month feed organ meat eg raw liver. Throughout the week natural cottage cheese, goats milk, cooked eggs or if raw egg yolk only can be feed without any problems.

**30% Vegies** - (anything green or yellow) eg 1/2 teaspoon mixed into daily meals.. If cooked best to use pumpkin well mashed if uncooked well mulched carrot and or zucchini.

**10% Herbs** - Add daily about 1 tablespoon of finely chopped parsley (cleanses kidneys of toxins) and garlic finely chopped or minced into meals, quarter clove for pets under 5kg, 1 clove for 10 to 30kg.

**Note -** Cats need more calories than dogs and more saturated fat but require fewer carbohydrates and less roughage. Cats also do not need as much minerals as humans and dogs need.

Fish and tuna oils can deplete animals of Vit E which can in turn cause steatitis.

# Supplements for the Cat
## Vitamin and Mineral Powder for Cats
### Mix the powder supplements together and store in a air tight container

1. 1/4 cup of bone meal or Dolomite
2. 1/4 Cup of Kelp Powder
3. 1/8 Cup of Lecithin grains
4. Add a pinch of **vitamin C** in the form of Ester C powder. (for general health maintenance and as a antioxidant).
5. Add daily a quarter teaspoon full to every meal eg am and pm meals. (start off by only adding a pinch full at a time till the cat gets used to it).

## Other Supplements

**Sesame seed oil cold pressed** - supplies EFAs. Dosage 1/8 to 1/4 teaspoon - mix well into food.

**B - Complex -** 50 to 70mg can be given to animals that are stressed, nervous or are recovering from surgery or injury. Also give for behaviour disorder - chewing, hyperactivity etc., crush tablet and add to meals. Brewer's yeast is a good source of the B vitamins

**Barley Green Powder** - Can be added to meals for extra nutrition especially when the pet is sick or unwell. Add 3 teaspoons to meals.

**Evening Primrose Oil -** is vital to the immune system and contains GLA, Vit E and omega 6 and 9. Good for pets suffering from arthritis, skin disease, hormone problems and bone degenerative diseases. Add 1 teaspoon to meals.

**Cod liver oil -** Supplies Vitamins A and D, give half a teaspoon twice weekly mixed with Evening Primrose Oil.

**Notes**

1.  Avoid overfeeding.
2.  Avoid a exclusive diet of any one food. Offer different foods so the cat learns to accept variety.
3.  Milk after the kitten stage may provoke diarrhea.
4.  Avoid chocolate as this can cause seizures.
5.  Dog food is not suitable for cats.
6.  Meals should be a specific amount left out for twenty to thirty minutes and then cleared away.
7.  Animal protein is essential for cats for this contains the essential amino acid Taurine which cats can't manufacture for themselves and must get from the diet. Deficiencies can lead to blindness.
8.  Cats must have essential fatty acids found in vegetable oils. Without them a cats coat loses its shine and reproductive disorders may occur.
9.  A comprehensive range of vitamins and minerals needs to be present in your cat's diet. This is particularly true of Vitamin A since cats are unable to use carotenes to manufacture it.

# How to Take a Cats Temperature

A cat's normal temperature is between 38.1 and 39.2 degrees Celsius (100.5 to 102.5 F). Nervousness and exercise raise the bodies temperature as do excess heat and infections. Temperatures below normal are caused by exposure to cold weather but can also be caused by shock. Make a note of your cat's normal body temperature when he it is at rest so you have a good comparison when something is wrong.

1.  If using a glass thermometer, shake it down, lubricate the tip with K-Y jelly and using a slight rotating action insert it about 2.5 cm into the cat's rectum. This is more a job for two people with one holding the cat and the other taking the temperature.

2.  Keep hold of the thermometer and the cat's tail, wait for about 90 seconds and then remove, wipe clean and read. Disinfect the thermometer after each use.



## Temperature Range

**41.1+C or 106+ F-** Cool cat down and go to Vets immediately
**40.6C or 105 F-** Take to the Vet today
**40C or 104F –** Fever
**39.4C or 103F -** Fever
**38.9C or 102F -** Normal
**38.3C or101 –** Normal
**37.8C or 101F -** Normal to onset of mild hypothermia
**37.2C or 99 -** See vet today
**36.7C or 98F -** Keep cat warm take to vet immediately

# Diseases of the Respiratory System
## Signs and Symptoms

## Coughing

Generally this is associated with respiratory infections or obstructions of the airways. A cough is a reflex action brought on by irritation of the air passages.

Things to look for.

1.  Is something stuck in the throat.
2.  Are there any typical cold and flu signs such as fever, breathing problems, nasal or eye discharges, sneezing?
3.  Is the cat bringing up any phlegm, if so it may have an acute chest infection.
4.  Does the cough sound bubbly, if so fluid may of built up in the chest from a infection.
5.  Does the cough sound dry and hacking if so the cat may have acute bronchitis.
6.  Are there any pollutants in the air that may be causing the irritation. (allergic reaction).

## Panting

At rest a cat takes 25 to 30 breaths a minute. After exercise this rises to 60 to 90. If you think your cat is breathing rapidly count the rate.

Things to look for

1.  Is the weather very hot, the cat may be just trying to cool down.
2.  Are the cats nostrils obstructed, a blockage may be preventing it from breathing properly.
3.  Is there any sign of a accident, the cat may have a chest or lung injury or maybe shock.
4.  Has the cat been in a fight check for the above.
5.  Are there any signs of a respiratory disease such as fever, coughing, nasal or eye discharge or sneezing present.

## Shallow Breathing

A cat will only breathe shallowly if breathing deeply causes pain.

Things to look for

1.   Has the cat been in a accident causing damage to the chest area.

2.   Has the cat lost its appetite, it may have a severe viral infection.(pleurisy)

3.   Are the lip, tongue and gums gray or blue as this occurs when there is insufficient oxygen in the blood.

## Sneezing

Generally associated with respiratory infections, sneezing is a reflex action brought on by irritation of the nasal passages.

Things to look for

1.   Has the cat a nasal discharge, if so it is probably a infection.

2.   Are there any cold or flu signs present, fever, breathing problems, nasal or eye discharges, coughing.

Possible causes may be bacterial or fungal infection of the nostril or sinuses, a virus, allergic reaction, or at worst a nasal tumour.

## Wheezing

A whistling sound made on exhalation or inhalation, wheezing is a result of a partial obstruction at some point between the larynx and the bronchioles. This narrows the tube producing the sound.

Things to look for

1.   Are the cats lips tongue and gums grey or blue in colour. This occurs when there is insufficient oxygen in the blood. It may indicate a heart problem.

2.   Coughing - this might indicate the presence of lung worm.

Possible causes may be asthma, lung worm, congestive heart failure or maybe a tumour in the air passages.

## Overview for the Respiratory System

**For most conditions of the respiratory system Echinacea and Garlic (very small doses) should be very seriously considered especially if the condition is a result of bacteria or viruses and even if it is not they should still be considered as a preventative for secondary infections. Doses of Vitamin C are also very important to consider. Licorice is another good herb for the respiratory system as some of its actions are expectorant and demulcent but the main reason I am**

mentioning it is that you usually add liquorice (Not To Be Used In Patients With High Blood Pressure) to a herbal formula so as to help the body of the patient to absorb the formula. Try not to use more than five herbs in a formula and use the actions you require to select the herbs, you can do this easily by using my First Aid For Animals Booklet by accessing the Herbal and Actions section.

## Upper Respiratory Problems

Cats seem to have similar problems as do humans, coughing, sneezing, watery nose and eyes, looking rotten and breathing changes. Often these problems are a sign of a mild illness that will clear up in a few days with careful nursing. However these can also be signs of a more severe or fatal illness especially if there is fever, loss of appetite, listlessness and dehydration.

## Viral Diseases

Cats have their own types of respiratory viruses that can range from mild to fatal; the two below are the most dangerous out of the flu like ones.

## Feline Rhinotracheitis (Herpes virus)

Symptoms are sneezing, coughing, eyes and nose discharge, fever, drooling, lack of appetite, termination of pregnancy (abortion). Has a 2 to 10 day incubation period after this it produces inflammation of the eyes, nose, and windpipe along with the resultant discharges. The Cat becomes apathetic and feverish, loses its appetite and sneezes continually. Discharges from eyes and nose become thicker and purulent and sometimes the cat develops painful ulcers on its tongue. This is usually a severe infection of longer then a week's duration and can be fatal especially to kittens and the elderly cat. Recovered animals can become carriers.

For more information see this heading in the chapter on Infectious Diseases.

## Feline Calici Virus

Symptoms - The incubation period is about 5 to 7 days, temperature rise, followed by lethargy, poor appetite, watery discharge from the eyes and nose and dribbling from the mouth, ulcers on the tongue. Recovery normally takes place in a week. Infection can be from very mild to fatal. Good nursing is very important, clean away discharge from eyes and nose. Inhalations may help with breathing.
For more information see this heading in the chapter on Infectious Diseases.

## Feline Influenza (Picornavirus)

Symptoms - Sneezing, eye discharge, lack of appetite, fever, ulcers on tongue, drooling. There are more than 15 different strains of this. Symptoms vary from mild to severe. Recovered cats may become carriers. With this condition try and treat the symptoms, get your information from other headings in this chapter.

# Rhinitis

This means inflammation of the nasal mucous membranes and it usually occurs as part of another problem, often cat flu. Inflammation is started by something irritating the linings of the mucous membranes and after this has been established for a while opportunistic infectious agents usually try to take advantage of the situation with the main culprits being Staphylococcal and Streptococci Bacteria.

## Signs and Symptoms

Nasal discharge is a constant sign which usually starts clear and thin and then changes in stages becoming muco-purulent. Streaks of blood may be present. There is usually bouts of sneezing along with the discharge. The discharge may be acrid in which case the nostrils may be inflamed and sore. Persistent discharges may impede the breathing by blocking up a nostril. Where the discharge is from one nostril only and not a foreign body, it could be a fungal infection, usually Asoergillus. In this condition the discharge will be thick and green and may persist for a long time, even months.

## Herbal Treatment

Herbs to look at here besides the overview ones can be Eye Bright, Golden Rod, Sage, Thyme and Elder Flowers. Anti-fungal herbs to think of are Calendula, Sweet Violets.

## Homoeopathic Treatment

**Arsenic Album 30C**- For the early stages when the discharge is thin and acrid, eyes may be watery and patient is thirsty for small quantities of water. The coat may be dry and harsh and symptoms may get worse towards midnight. Try one dose daily for ten days.

**Pulsatilla 30C**- Mild tempered animals showing changeable moods, discharge is thick ,creamy and bland ,there may be ulceration of the nostrils with small streaks of blood. Try one dose daily for up to seven days.

**Mercurius Sol 6C** - Greenish discharge, may contain blood, nasal bones are frequently swollen, symptoms are worse from sunset to sunrise. Give three times daily for seven days.

**Allium Cepa 6C** - Discharges are usually thin and watery accompanied by sneezing and watery eyes, useful in the first stages. Give one dose three times daily for three days.

**Kali Bich 30C** - Yellow discharges which develop into small plugs which have a tough stringy appearance. Streaks of blood are often present. Give one dose daily for ten days.

# Sinusitis

These occasionally become infected or inflamed resulting in a collection of purulent material in the area. The pain is usually from the pressure the expanding mucous puts on the surrounding area. Infection usually spreads from other areas with a common cause being a infected tooth.

The condition can lead to nasal discharges of a offensive nature which can be difficult to treat.

## Signs and Symptoms

Infection of a frontal sinus usually results in a purulent nasal discharge which may become streaked with blood. There is usually accompanying conjunctivitis. As for any health problem try to remove the cause, in this case it could be a infected tooth.

## Herbal Treatment

Herbs to look at here besides the ones mentioned in the overview are Ginger and Cayenne which are warm spicy circulatory stimulants which act by thinning the mucous and are called mucotropic. If either of these herbs is used they can replace the liquorice in the formula for circulatory stimulants are used for getting the formula into the system as well. Other herbs to consider are Fenugreek, Eye Bright, Horse Radish (mucotropic) and Golden Rod.

## Homoeopathic Treatment

**Hepar Sulph 6C** - Indicated where there is pain and sensitivity over the affected area. Low potencies will promote expulsion of any residual pus while high potencies will provide healing by granulation. Three times daily for lower potencies and three times per week for four weeks for the higher potencies eg 200.

**Silicea 200C** - For long standing cases where symptoms are less sensitive. It will help the healing process by drying any discharge and removing scar tissue. Give one dose 3 times weekly for 4 weeks.

# Tonsillitis

Inflammation of the tonsils is a fairly common occurrence and can be either chronic or acute. The effected tissue becomes swollen and reddened due to increased blood supply and may show small greyish spots of necrosis and frothy exudate. Appetite may be variable and there is discomfort on swallowing. Reaching is a frequent accompaniment with vomiting of any excess mucous. A rise of temperature is usual in the early stages especially in kittens.

## Herbal Treatment

Herbs to look at here besides the ones mentioned in the overview are Poke Root (use in very small doses or the Homoeopathic dose see Phytolacca 30C below), Myrrh, Mullein, Sage, Thyme and Cleavers.

## Homoeopathic Treatment

**Acute Form**

**Aconitum 30C** - Give as early as possible where it can sometimes stop the problem from developing further.

**Belladonna 30C** - A useful remedy along with Aconitum in the early stages. The patient may show excitability with dilated pupils and a full throbbing pulse along with a raised temperature.

**Phytolacca 30C** - Where the tonsils are enlarged and the throat has a dark red colour. Membranous deposits may be present along with yellowish mucous. Give one dose twice daily for seven days.

**Rhus Tox 6C** - The throat shows large amounts of mucous and assumes a unnatural reddish colour. Externally the throat may be swollen. There may be accompanying eye symptoms.

**Apis 6C** - Excessive oedema of tonsillar tissue, warm drinks aggravate.

**Lachesis 12C** - The tonsillar tissue appears dark bluish red or purple and considerable swelling is present. The condition appears to be aggravated after sleep. Give one dose three times daily for five days.

**Chronic Form**

This can be a sequel to some disease in the past that has not left the system yet. The following remedies will be of help.

**Silicea 200C** - Promotes the absorption of any fibrous or scar tissue which may be present and will control and tendency to suppuration. Give one dose twice weekly for seven weeks.

**Baryta Carb - 6C** - Both very young and old subjects will benefit from this remedy. There is a marked tendency to suppuration of the tonsillar tissue. Give one dose three times daily for 5 days.

**Hepar Sulph 30C** - Tonsils which periodically show purulent infection may be helped by this remedy. The throat becomes extremely painful and sensitive to pressure during acute episodes. Give one dose daily for ten days.

**Kali Bich 200C** - Swollen tonsils becoming ulcerated and yielding a stringy yellow pus, the tissue assumes a reddish coppery tinge. Give one dose twice daily for six weeks.

**Streptococcus Nosode 30C** - This nosode can be combined with the above remedies.

Give one dose daily for five days.

# Laryngitis

Inflammation of the larynx may be acute or chronic. The acute form is usually associated with primary infection or having spread from another area. There are varying degrees of severity encountered some proving fatal by blocking off the airway.

## Signs and Symptoms

The owner's attention is first alerted by the cat making gulping noises as though some obstruction were present. There is a loss of voice or a change in its character. Pressure over the laryngeal area is resented and in some cases there is extreme difficulty in breathing with the mouth being kept open.

## Herbal Treatment

Herbs to look at here besides the ones mentioned in the overview are Mullein (demulcent), Sage, Elder Flowers, Golden Rod  and have a look at Plantain.

## Homoeopathic Treatment

### Acute Form

**Aconitum 30C** - Give as early as possible where it can sometimes stop the problem from developing further.

**Belladonna 12C** - Indicated for the animal which shows excitability, full bounding pulse and dilated pupils, can be profitably combined with the above remedy. Give one dose every hour for four doses.

**Apis 30C** - Much oedema and throat swelling, aversion to warmth of any kind and is thirstless. Give one dose three times daily for three days.

**Spongia 6C -** Indicated in laryngeal conditions attended by a hoarse croupous cough, there is a absence of mucous, there may be whistling with the respiration. One dose three times daily for seven days.

**Drosera 9C** - Spasmodic cough associated with the upper trachea and larynx, hoarseness is very pronounced, there is also tenacious mucous, the cough usually produces reaching and vomiting in the cat and greatly impedes breathing. One dose three times daily for seven days.

**Causticum 30C** - Indicated in those cases where the voice becomes lost due to a temporary paralysis of the laryngeal nerves. The cough may cause urination, mucous gathers in the throat with great difficulty expelling it. Give one dose twice daily for ten days.

**Rhus Tox 1M** - Indicated when the larynx is deep red and the cough is attended by greenish mucous of a putrid nature, occasionally blood is present. A generalized stiffness of movement may be present. Give one dose daily for twelve days.

# Bronchitis

Usually indicated by a cough and is caused by inflammation of the lining of the air tubes (bronchi) that link the wind pipe to the lungs. This leads to excess mucous being produced which reduces the space in the airways.  Causes can be irritants such as smoke, foreign bodies or infections.

There is a seasonal association  in connection with this trouble. The chief symptom is coughing which can vary in severity. Rattling sounds may sometimes be heard. Appetite is maintained and there is little or no fever. If this problem keeps recurring it can lead to permanent damage of the respiratory system. Some cats that live with smokers develop Chronic Bronchitis. Older cats are more prone to Chronic Bronchitis with obesity increasing the odds.

## Signs and Symptoms

Persistent coughing or coughing bouts that keeps recurring where mucous is coughed up by the cat. Exercise or normal effort can cause rapid exhaustion and a increase in the breathing rate. An x-ray is usually used for diagnosis. This disease can make the body ripe for a infection so be very careful.

## Herbal Treatment

Herbs to look at here besides the ones mentioned in the overview are Mullein and Plantain, as demulcents they will ease the pain if the area is dry, if there is lots of mucous we need to use astringents to slow the flow may be Eye Bright and Elecampane (anti-bacterial to) other herbs to look at are Fenugreek, Coltsfoot, Golden Rod ,Liquorice, Grindelia , Hyssop and Horehound with the last two being good for the cough. Steamers (humidifier) or a room full of Eucalyptus steam may help with breathing. Eucalyptus oil is a Bronchodilator. Consider also Vitamin C.

## Homoeopathic Treatment

**Byronia 6C -** This remedy is indicated when the animal is better resting, pressure over the affected area gives relief,

**Kali Bich 200C -** Where mucous of a stringy yellow nature is expectorated, there may be a accompanying nasal discharge. Give one dose three times per week for four weeks.

**Antimonium Tart 30C -** Rattling of mucous is a prominent symptom, the discharge being frothy and mucoid

**Apis Mel 6C -** When excess fluid is suspected leading to expectoration of fluid mucous this remedy may help.

**Spongia 6C -** Useful remedy in the older animal where there are accompanying symptoms of heart involvement.

# Bronchiectasis

This is where the bronchial tree becomes abnormally dilated due to a loss of tone or elasticity in its fibers. This allows fluid to develop in pockets which eventually become pockets for purulent material. This condition is frequently a sequel to some other pulmonary disease but it can also arise as a result of a foreign body being breathed into the lung.

## Signs and Symptoms

Continual coughing which is dry and unproductive in the early stages but soon becomes moist and the patient coughs up large quantities of mucopurulent material.

## Herbal Treatment

Herbs to look at here besides the ones mentioned in the overview are Elecampane, Ginger, Red Clover. If there is lots of mucous we need to use astringents to slow the flow may be Eye Bright and Elecampane (anti-bacterial to) other herbs to look at are Fenugreek, Coltsfoot, Golden Rod ,Liquorice, Hyssop and Horehound with the last two being good for the cough. With this being a long term condition use Echinacea on a month on month off basis so as not to burn out the immune system.

## Homoeopathic Treatment

**Bryonia 6C -** May help in the early dry and unproductive stage, the animal resents movement and pressure over the chest gives relief.

**Antimonium Tart 30C -** A useful remedy in the early stages when the cough is attended with frothy exudate. Rattling of mucous in the airways is a prominent symptom.

**Hepar Sulph 30C -** A good remedy in the early purulent stages and will limit the risk of secondary bacterial involvement.

**Kali Bich 30C -** Indicated when the cough is accompanied by tough mucous of a yellow stringy nature.

**Merc Sol 6C -** This remedy could be indicated when any material coughed up is of a greenish rather than of a yellow colour.

# Diseases of the Lungs and Pleura

## Pulmonary Oedema

The abnormal accumulation of fluid in the lung is usually a sequel to chronic heart disease, especially mitral valve insufficiency which causes weak circulation and allows fluid to gather in other areas especially the lungs.

## Signs and Symptoms

There is great difficulty in breathing and a moist cough is fairly constant. If it accompanies some other disease signs of this will be present also.

## Herbal Treatment

If this condition is caused by a failing heart the herbs to look at here are Hawthorn and Broom but if it is from a infection use the herbs in the overview.

## Homoeopathic Treatment

**Apis 30C -** This remedy is always indicated when oedema is present and should aid in resorption.

**Strophanthus 3X -** This heart remedy is indicated as it stimulates the heart action and will hasten output of urine and thereby help to reduce the fluid. Give one dose twice daily for 30 days.

**Cactus Grandiflourus 6C -** This is a good heart remedy which will stimulate the hearts action and thereby increase circulation.

**Adonis Vernalis 6C** - This is also a good heart remedy which should have a beneficial effect in valvular disease.

**Crataegus 6C** - A heart remedy which exerts its action on the muscle thereby increasing the force of the beat and the flow of the circulation.

**Carbo Veg 30C** - Gives relief by helping the patient's oxygen supply and thereby aiding breathing in general.

# Emphysema

When the alveoli of the lungs loose their elasticity becoming distended and unable to return to their normal size a state of emphysema is said to exist. In severe cases the alveolar wall may rupture permitting the escape of air into surrounding tissues. This condition is usually caused or is the end result of other diseases with a good example being pneumonia.

## Signs and Symptoms

There is obvious difficulty in expelling air and respiration may be associated with forced movements of the abdominal muscles in order to assist the process. There is general difficulty in breathing. Tension in the pulmonary vessels arise as a result of increased pressure on the right ventricle of the heart.

## Herbal Treatment

This is a long term chronic disease and treatment would be similar to what is mentioned in Bronchiectasis with the addition of Coltsfoot. Panax Ginseng Capsules (divide capsules in quarters and give 4 times a day so the cat is only getting one capsule a day) could be useful by raising the life force and helping the patient to get the best out of their condition. Ginseng is used 1 month on and one month off otherwise it can over stimulate.

## Homoeopathic Treatment

These remedies will work at the onset of the condition but will not be much help in the chronic condition.

**Acconitum 6C** - Always indicated where there is tension in any part of the circulatory system and should give relief indirectly as a result.

**Lobellia 30C** - Useful in the treatment of functional emphysema where the changes in the alveolar walls have not gone too far or become chronic.

**Carbo Veg 30C** - Will provide oxygen by its ability to help in cases of air hunger; will give relief particularly at night.

# Pneumonia

Inflammation of the lung with exudation and consolidation. Pneumonia is not common in cats and is generally a complication of other diseases such as a severe flu, bacterial or fungal infection, lung worms or an inhalation of liquids. Rehydradition is a very important in this condition. A vet would use an x-ray to confirm diagnosis.

## Signs and Symptoms

There is a initial rise in temperature. The cat looks anxious with respirations increased and in severe cases painful breathing is evident and may have a tendency to stay still. Coughing may be a fairly constant sign along with coughing up large amounts of phlegm and mucous. The animal becomes dehydrated and unkempt and water intake is decreased. A cat affected with Pneumonia will typically stand with their front legs spread and head lowered, often coughing and trying to take in more air.

## Herbal Treatment

Herbs to look at here besides the ones mentioned in the overview are Golden Rod, Ginger and Peppermint for the fever, Mullein, Elecampane and Horehound for the cough, other useful herbs are Golden Rod, Elder ,Coltsfoot, Hyssop, Sage, Thyme and Plantain. Garlic is a very important herb here as it exits the body mostly via the lungs and its actions would be felt as it was leaving.

## Homoeopathic Treatment

The following remedies may help if the symptoms match.

**Aconitum 6C** - Give as early as possible where it can sometimes stop the problem from developing further.

**Antimonium Tart 30C** - Where there is a abundance of loose mucous and expectoration.

**Bryonia 6C** - When this remedy is indicated the animal resents movement, pressure over the affected area bring relief, the animal prefers to lie on the effected side. Better from rest.

**Ferrum Phos 12C** - The animal may show signs of pain and anxiety when breathing in. There is a abundance of loose mucous in the throat. Coughing may produce blood and is associated with blood.

**Phosphorus 30C -** Expectoration of rust coloured sputum associated with rapid breathing. Alternatively the cough may be dry and unproductive. A good remedy for the nervous and sensitive.

# Pleurisy

Inflammation of the pleural membranes can be either dry or accompanied by effusion into the pleural sack. The cause is usually from the spread of infection from another part of the respiratory system. Fairly common in cats, pleurisy is a build-up of milky white liquid in the chest cavity that compresses the lung and makes breathing difficult.

## Signs and Symptoms

The animal appears anxious and there are signs of abdominal breathing signifying pain on inspiration. If one side only is effected the animal seeks to lie on that side while if the animal assumes a sitting position it usually indicates both sides are effected. The temperature may rise to 105 F and accompanies early signs of pain.

## Herbal Treatment

Herbs to look at here besides the ones mentioned in the overview are Peppermint and Ginger for any fever, and other useful herbs are Golden Rod, Hyssop, Horehound, Yarrow, Coltsfoot and Elder. Garlic would be a good remedy for this condition.

## Homoeopathic treatment

**Acconitum 30C** - Should always be given as early in the condition as possible, as it will quickly allay anxiety and helps to relieve pain.

**Belladonna 30C -** A useful remedy if the animal feels unduly hot with dilated pupils and throbbing pulse and displays nervous symptoms or is excitable.

**Bryonia 6C or 30C** - This is probably the best remedy to consider in most cases once the condition has established. A main guiding principle for its use is relief of pain on pressure seen by the animal lying on the effected side and disinclined to move.

**Apis 30C** - This remedy should help to reduce the fluid which is present in those cases showing effusion and may also help with the pain.

# Herbal Overview of the Respiratory System

For most conditions of the respiratory system Echinacea and Garlic should be very seriously considered especially if the condition is a result of bacteria or viruses and even if it is not they should still be considered as a preventative for secondary infections. Doses of Vitamin C are also very important to consider. Liquorice is another good herb for the respiratory system as some of its actions are expectorant and demulcent but the main reason I am mentioning it is that you usually add liquorice to a herbal formula so as to help the body of the patient to absorb the formula. Try not to use more than five herbs in a formula and use the actions you require to select the herbs, you can do this easily by using my First Aid For Animals Booklet by accessing the Herbal and Actions section.

Below are the Actions to think of when dealing with the Respiratory System. As usual isolate the animal and observe. Consider also if the condition is affecting another system. Is there diarrhea, is there any unusual behaviour, is there fever, what is the temperature, is the animal anxious etc. Some of the best herbs for this system are Angelica, Coltsfoot, Comfrey, Elder, Elecampane, Eyebright, Fenugreek, Golden Rod, Hyssop, Horehound, Horse Radish, Liquorice, Mullein, Myrrh, Plantain, Sage and Thyme.

## Herbal Actions for the Respiratory System

**Anti-biotic** - Echinacea, Elecampane, Garlic, Burdock, Myrrh.

**Anti-catarrhal** - Helps the body to remove excess catarrhal build ups.

**Herbs** - Cayenne, Coltsfoot, Cranesbill, Echinacea, Elder, Eyebright, Garlic, Golden Rod, Hyssop, Marshmallow, Mullein, Myrrh, Peppermint, Sage, Thyme, Yarrow.

**Anti-inflammatory -** Helps the body to combat inflammations. Herbs mentioned under demulcents will often act in this way especially when they coat sore throats and pipe lines.

**Herbs** - Comfrey, Cranesbill, Eyebright, Feverfew, Ginger, Golden Rod, Lady's Mantle, Licorice, Marshmallow.

**Anti-microbial** - Helps the body destroy or resist pathogenic micro-organisms.

**Herbs** - Aniseed, Echinacea, Garlic, Myrrh, Peppermint, Plantain, Rosemary, Sage, Thyme.

**Antispasmodic** - Prevents or eases spasms and cramps.

**Herbs** - Aniseed, Coltsfoot, Fennel, Horehound, Hyssop, Mullein, Rosemary, Sage, Skullcap, Thyme

**Anti-viral** - Astragalus, Echinacea, Elecampane, Garlic, Myrrh?, Shitake, St John's Wort, Pau D'Arco.

**Anthelmintic** - Destroys or expels worms from the digestive system.

**Herbs** - Garlic, Tansy, Wormwood, Thyme, Rue.

**Astringent** - Contracts tissue which in turn reduces discharges, these herbs contain tannins.

**Herbs** - Agrimony, Comfrey, Elecampane, Eyebright, Golden Rod, Marshmallow, Mullein, Myrrh, Plantain, Sage, Rosemary, Shepherds Purse, Thyme.

**Demulcent** - Soothes and protects irritated or inflamed internal tissues.

**Herbs** - Coltsfoot, Comfrey, Fenugreek, Liquorice, Marshmallow, Mullein, Oats, Plantain.

**Diaphoretic** - Aids the skin in the elimination of toxins and produces sweat thus reducing the temperature of fevers.

**Herbs** - Cayenne, Elder, Elecampane, Fennel, Garlic, Ginger, Golden Rod, Hyssop, Peppermint, Thyme, Yarrow.

**Expectorant** - Supports the body in the removal of excess mucous from the respiratory system and helps in the control of coughs.

**Herbs** - Aniseed, Coltsfoot, Comfrey, Elder, Elecampane, Fennel, Fenugreek, Garlic, Hyssop, Horehound, Liquorice, Marshmallow, Mullein, Myrrh, Plantain, Sweet Violets, Thyme.

**Febrifuge** - Helps the body to bring down fevers.

**Herbs** - Cayenne, Elder Flowers, Hyssop, Marigold, Penny Royal, Peppermint, Plantain, Raspberry, Sage, Thyme, Vervain.

**Immune Booster** - Astragalus, Echinacea, Reshi, Shitake.

**Pectoral** - Has a general strengthening and healing effect on the respiratory system.

**Herbs** - Aniseed, Coltsfoot, Comfrey, Elder, Garlic, Hyssop, Licorice, Mullein, Horehound.

# The Digestive System

## Diarrhoea

Can be a natural way for the body to remove toxins. This is sometimes accompanied by vomiting. Long lasting diarrhoea or bloody diarrhoea should be taken to the vet. Causes can be a bacterial or viral infection, parasites especially in kittens, food allergies (milk), diet especially all meat diets, hypermotility (bowel moving too fast), stress or may be a more serious disease such as Feline Infectious Peritonitis.

**Symptoms** - loose faeces, abdominal straining with maybe abdominal pain and there may be some dehydration.

## Different Types

1.  **Hypermotility** - Bowel is moving too fast. – The stools can be green to yellow and watery, the smell may be a little strong or sour. Causes can be Irritant Chemicals, heavy worm burden, stagnant water, rotting food, bacterial toxins, rich or very fatty foods
2.  **Malabsorption** - Food not being digested properly – The stools can be pale grey to yellow and look greasy. Causes can be liver or pancreas conditions, indigestible foods, over eating, internal parasites.
3.  **Infection** - Bacterial, Viral or infection from parasite. – The stools can vary but may be very fluid and may have gas bubbles. The smell is usually offensive and the frequency can be up to several times a hour.  Causes can be bacterial or viral infections, poisons, drugs

**Notes**

1.  There are some agents such as internal parasites that could directly or indirectly cause any of the 3 types of bowel problems.
2.  The severity depends on the degree of the insult
3.  The overall health of the cat must also be considered. In very young or old cats or in debilitated cats diarrhoea is always a significant sign and potentially serious.

**See Vet if diarrhoea is accompanied by vomiting**

## Herbal Treatment

**Diarrhoea -** This is a method the body uses to get rid of toxins that are aggravating it so it is best to let it run its course and be on the watch for dehydration and take steps to prevent this from happening. Some people give laxatives with this condition so as to try to clear the toxins out fast. Always try to find the cause of the problem, is it diet, stress, allergies, gastritis is a common cause for diarrhoea followed by worm infestations or it could be part of a symptom picture of a infectious disease. The cat should be fasted till the condition improves or for 24 hours at least. Diarrhoea is usually treated with astringents usually the milder ones as the very strong ones may upset a sensitive tummy. Some examples are Agrimony and Slippery Elm which is the best for recovery as it is demulcent and nutritive. If a infectious type of disease is suspected add Garlic (very small quantities) and Echinacea.

## Homoeopathic Treatment

**Arsenic Alb 6 of 30C** - This remedy is associated with watery stools of a cadaverous odour frequently worse in the evenings and towards midnight. Thirst for small amounts of water, the coat is harsh and dry and the patient is restless changing position from time to time, a good remedy when there are signs of dehydration.

**Ipecac 30C** - Indicated when severe vomiting precedes a attack, frequent mucous like stools which are greenish in colour and may also be tinged with blood.

**Podophyllum 30C** - Remedy for conditions affecting both small and large intestines resulting in a gushing type of watery stool that may contain mucous. It is suitable for long standing diarrhoea and may be accompanied by a degree of rectal prolapse.

**Pulsatilla 30C** - For yellow stool particularly if the consistency changes from stool to stool and the cat complains.

**Veratrum Alb 30C** - Prostration accompanies the diarrhoea and there is a general picture of collapse, signs of colic precede the onset of diarrhea which is profuse and watery. General signs include a dry mouth and cyanosis of visible mucous membranes.

**Cuprum Met 30C** - Muscular cramping may be seen accompanying diarrhea of a greenish blood stained character. Nervous symptoms are often present e.g twitching.

**Carbo Veg 200C** - A most useful remedy for the dead looking animal and will frequently give dramatic results in apparently hopeless cases which have suffered severe fluid loss. The stools have a cadaverous odour and are attended with considerable wind.

**China 6C -** This remedy should always be given as a accompaniment to others as it will help restore health after loss of body fluid, by itself it may control the diarrhoea.

# Constipation

A healthy cat usually opens it bowels once or twice a day. Difficulty in passing stools can be from obstruction or from the stools being to hard. Attention must be paid to the diet assuring that plenty of bulk is available in the food together with a proper fluid intake.

## Things to look for

1.   Are the stools hard and dark? This indicates a lack of fluid present.
2.   Is the cat straining and not passing stools? If normal stools are present it may be a urinary tract infection.
3.   Is the diet correct?
4.   If the cat is a long haired cat fur balls could be causing the condition.
5.   If the cat is vomiting there may be a serious intestinal blockage.
6.   Old age leads to weaker abdominal muscles.

**Constipation -** Can be mild or severe and has its origin in reduced fluid intake, lack of bulk or sometimes just age. The first place to start is to look at the diet.

Laxative herbs are Burdock, Dandelion, Liquorice, Fumitory and Horseradish. Stronger ones are Cascara and Senna Pods. Always buffer with a demulcent herb to stop bad side effects.

## Homoeopathic Treatment

**Nux Vom 6C -** For digestive disturbances generally, There is frequent straining with passage of small amounts at a time. The origin of the trouble is usually dietary upset and may be associated with vomiting. This is a good digestive remedy and will help regulate proper bowel movements.

**Sulphur 6C -** Usually pronounced redness around the anus accompanied by much scratching in general, body odour may be musty, acts well with Nux Vom.

**Carbo Veg 30C -** You can give this if your cat is suffering indigestion after eatting a rich meal. Good for gas and general indigestion problems.

**Bryonia 6C -** Stools are large and dark coloured (may have a burnt look) and passed more frequently in the morning, the animal is generally uneasy and is disinclined to move, listless. Tenderness over the abdomen is very pronounced although pressure is not resented. The cat is thirsty and irritable.

**Lycopodium 1M -** Usually a history of liver problems or accompanying hepatitis. Stools are small and the appetite is capricious, very little satisfying. Lean or undernourished looking animals may respond well to this remedy with other symptoms agreeing, worse in the afternoon.

**Plumbum 30C -** Give this if your cat has hard black stools.


# Flatulence

This condition is caused by undigested carbohydrates which when fermented by bacteria in the colon produce gas.

### Things to look for

1. What is the diet like.
2. Is the problem constantly present, if so it is likely to be caused by a absorption problem.
3. Do the droppings look normal.

**Carbo Veg 30C -** You can give this if your cat is suffering indigestion after eating a rich meal. Good for gas and general indigestion problems.


# Gastritis and Vomiting

Means inflammation of the stomach. In cats trouble of this nature is usually due to impaction of fur balls or furry material which the animal has been unable to expel in the normal way. Other irritants can cause this condition also.

### Signs and Symptoms

The cat exhibits signs of uneasiness and attempts may be made to vomit. The condition is relatively mild in cats. Gastritis due to ingestion of foreign material may occur occasionally but is less likely in this species then in the dog. A bout of occasional vomiting, for example bringing up hairballs in a otherwise healthy cat is generally not a cause for concern. If it is persistent however with or without other symptoms further investigation is needed. Vomiting causes dehydration so ensure plenty of water is available. Some causes can be from eating grass or foreign bodies, ingestion of poison, kidney failure, worms, hairballs, over eating or maybe a food sensitivity.

## Herbal Treatment

Marshmallow, Slippery Elm and Comfrey are soothing demulcent herbs which should line and sooth the raw areas. Other herbs to look at are Peppermint and Golden Rod..

### Homoeopathic treatment

**Nux Vom 6C -** A reliable remedy for simple indigestion and should stimulate the appetite, digestive disturbances generally, there may be vomiting flatulence and tenderness over the liver area.

**Arsenic Alb 30C -** For violent very frequent vomiting made worse by drinking cold water or vomiting.

**Phosphorus 30C -** Pronounced thirst but vomiting takes place as soon as the contents of the stomach become warm after drinking, gums may be ulcerated with slight bleeding, stools may be clay coloured, vomiting with pain. Useful remedy for nervous and sensitive animals

**Ipecacuanha 30C -** Retching and vomiting may lead to collapse. The vomit is slimy and may be continuous. Slimy diarrhoea possibly blood stained may be present also. There may also be reflex respiratory symptoms such as coughing and difficulty in breathing.

## Gastroenteritis

This is usually a mixture of vomiting and diarrhoea. The name means inflammation of the stomach and intestines. In a severe case you could see faecal matter in the vomit. Dehydration is a cause for concern here. Causes can range from food poisoning to a severe viral infection.

## Herbal Treatment

Similar to the section above and below with good herbs being Golden Rod, Marshmallow, Peppermint and slippery elm

**Homoeopathic Treatment**

Choose remedies from the section above and below Look especially at Arsenic and Ipecac.

# Enteritis and Colitis

Inflammatory conditions of the intestines results in diarrhoea and or dysentery with the character of the stool varying considerably. Acute episodes may arise as a result of bacterial attack or may be from specific diseases.

**Signs and Symptoms**

Vomiting may be seen initially but the main symptom is diarrhoea which at times may have blood in it. Temperature may arise if the attack is due to bacterial invasion but if poisoning is suspected the temperature will be normal. Pain is evident on abdominal palpation and rumbling of gut may be herd in the large bowel. Signs of dehydration appear if the diarrhoea is prolonged.

## Herbal Treatment

Slippery Elm should be thought of here not just for its soothing properties but because it is also astringent so it will help with diarrhoea, Comfrey has similar actions, Marshmallow is another demulcent. Other herbs to look at are Agrimony, Bayberry, Cranesbill (astringent), Fennel, Chamomile and Wild Yam for the inflammation and pain. Think of Echinacea and Garlic if you think the cause is from a infection.

## Homoeopathic Treatment

**Arsenic Alb 6 of 30C** - This remedy is associated with watery stools of a cadaverous odour frequently worse in the evenings and towards midnight. Thirst for small amounts of water, the coat is harsh and dry and the patient is restless changing position from time to time, a good remedy when there are signs of dehydration.

**Ipecac 30C** - Indicated when severe vomiting precedes a attack, frequent mucous like stools which are greenish in colour and may also be tinged with blood.

**Podophyllum 30C** - Remedy for conditions affecting both small and large intestines resulting in a gushing type of watery stool that may contain mucous. It is suitable for long standing diarrhoea and may be accompanied by a degree of rectal prolapse.

**Veratrum Alb 30C** - Prostration accompanies the diarrhoea and there is a general picture of collapse, signs of colic precede the onset of diarrhoea which is profuse and watery. General signs include a dry mouth and cyanosis of visible mucous membranes.

**Cuprum Met 30C** - Muscular cramping may be seen accompanying diarrhoea of a greenish blood stained character. Nervous symptoms are often present e.g twitching.

**China 6C -** This remedy should always be given as a accompaniment to others as it will help restore health after loss of body fluid, by itself it may control the diarrhoea.

## Food Allergies or Intolerances

Food allergy is a abnormal reaction to some ingredient in a food, quite frequently a protein. About one third of allergic reactions in cats are thought to be dietary triggered by such thing as cow's milk which a grown cat rarely needs. It is important to find the allergen and remove it from the diet. Common allergens are beef, dairy products such as milk or cheese, eggs, fish, chicken, grains such as wheat and corn, tofu or even snacks, maybe even flavoured vitamins.

**Symptoms** - bladder infections such as cystitis, digestive problems vomiting and or diarrhoea, itching can cause small scabs that look similar to flea allergy.

### Treatment

A elimination diet is the only way to find the offending allergen. Raw meat does not seem to cause the same allergic reaction as does cooked meat.

**Herbs -** Chamomile is a digestive herb that also has a anti-allergy effect. Peppermint is a nice gentle herb and also helps with pain.

**Vitamin C -** tablets may help to overcome symptoms of irritation since at high doses this vitamin acts as a natural antihistamine calming the bodies response to an allergen. Give 50mg up to 4 times a day.

# Diseases of the Liver

## Liver Problems

The liver is the largest internal organ and is most important to a cat. Its functions include the detoxification of drugs and chemicals, the elimination of toxins and waste products, the production of blood clotting factors, and the secretion of bile which is needed for digestion. The liver also stores fat soluble vitamins and iron. Because of the livers wide ranging tasks any interference with the way it works can cause wide ranging problems which can turn out to be very serious. One condition that can upset the liver is hepatitis which can come from a number of cause such as bacterial or viral infection, toxins or poisons. Fatty liver disease or hepatic lipidosis is an excessive accumulation of fat in the liver cells and is common in cats the cause is yet unknown.

## Treatment

Diet is the most important factor in treatment. A carefully controlled diet lessens the work of the liver allowing it time to recover, provide high value protein such as egg and offer the cat food in small amounts throughout the day. To stimulate the cats appetite try a mixture of honey and yoghurt. Raw liver given once a week supplies vitamins and iron. Vit C

## Signs and Symptoms

Symptoms of liver problems can be lack of appetite, weight loss and depression. Palpation over the right abdominal area may reveal a enlarged liver which is not always associated with pain. Vomiting and lack of appetite are usually present with liver problems.

The colour of the stool is a good guide to liver problems as the faeces can be grey or clay coloured. Jaundice is a sign that the liver is not functioning as it should and can usually be seen as a yellowish colour in the mucous membranes or the white parts of the eyes, with this sign there can also be bile in the urine giving it a yellowish greenish colour. In chronic disease and those associated with tumour formation abdominal dropsy is usually present.

## Herbal Treatment

With liver problems the best way to start would be a long fast so as to rest the liver and give it a chance to sort itself out.  Finding the cause is most important as if it is infection you will need to give Echinacea and Garlic to start on the battle with the causative agents.  Dandelion and Milk Thistle are two good herbs to look at for serious liver problems other herbs are Agrimony, Fumitory.

## Homoeopathic Treatment

This will depend on the overall symptom picture but there are certain remedies that have a action on the live and they include the following

**Chelidonium 6C** - Yellowish tongue and discoloration of visible mucous membranes, vomiting is usually present and signs of stiffness or pain may be evident over the right shoulder region, stools are clay coloured.

**Phosphorus 30C -** Vomiting is noticed shortly after animal takes food or water eg when it becomes warm in the stomach, small haemorrhages may be seen on the gums. With hepatitis the stools become pale and hard, the region over the liver becomes extremely tender on palpation.

**Aesculus 30C** - Jaundice, the portal circulation becomes congested leading to signs of abdominal discomfort soon after eating, tenderness over the liver, stools are large and hard and the urine becomes discoloured, there may be accompanying respiratory symptoms such as coughing up mucous.

**Lycopodium 1M**- A prominent liver remedy, inability to eat much at any one time, very little food appears to satisfy, all symptoms aggravated in the late afternoon and early evening, a good remedy for the old and for lean animals, premature greying of the coat could be another sign for this remedy, stools are generally hard.

**Nux Vom 1M** - If liver dysfunction is secondary to overeating or partaking of unsuitable food this remedy will be indicated. Stools are hard and the animal's temperament becomes uncertain.

**Sulphur 200C** - For liver disturbances in cats which show a dirty skin with redness of the skin around the anus and have a generally musty odour.

# Hepatitis

Inflammation of the liver may arise from time to time in cats. The patients usually have symptoms of bilious vomiting and of producing gray or coloured stools. Jaundice may or may not be present but if it is the stools may be a golden yellow. Poisons can cause Hepatitis.

## Herbal Treatment

Look at the herbs in the above section. If the Hepatitis is the infectious form use Echinacea and Garlic in your formula. If there is no infection just use Milk thistle by itself for a while.

## Homoeopathic Treatment

**Aconitum 30C** - Should be given as soon as possible, one dose every hour for four doses, use this remedy for the sudden onset of any acute disease.

**Phosphorus 30C** - Vomiting is noticed shortly after animal takes food or water eg when it becomes warm in the stomach, small haemorrhages may be seen on the gums. With hepatitis the stools become pale and hard, the region over the liver becomes extremely tender on palpation.

**Chelidonium 6C** - Yellowish tongue and discoloration of visible mucous membranes, vomiting is usually present and signs of stiffness or pain may be evident over the right shoulder region , stools are clay coloured.

**Lycopodium 12C** - A prominent liver remedy, inability to eat much at any one time, very little food appears to satisfy, all symptoms aggravated in the late afternoon and early evening, a good remedy for the old and for lean animals, premature greying of the coat could be another sign for this remedy, stools are generally hard. For the more chronic cases showing indigestion and flatulence.


# Cirrhosis of the Liver

The term implies a chronic thickening of the liver parenchyma leading to a hardening which can be felt on examination. It is of a fairly frequent occurrence in a cat.

## Signs and Symptoms

Symptoms include also constipation, vomiting and the presence large amounts of fluid in the abdominal cavity in severe cases. This arises from disturbances in the portal circulation.

## Herbal Treatment

Treatment is the same as is mentioned in liver problems. Milk Thistle is our best herb for the liver.

## Homoeopathic Treatment

**Phosphorus 200C** - Vomiting is noticed shortly after animal takes food or water eg when it becomes warm in the stomach, small haemorrhages may be seen on the gums. With hepatitis the stools become pale and hard, the region over the liver becomes extremely tender on palpation.

This remedy has a profound action on the liver. Give one dose twice weekly for four weeks.

**Lycopodium 200C** - Another valuable liver remedy for the older animal and one which shows a worsening of symptoms in late afternoon and early evening. Stools are usually dry and shiny. Give one dose three times weekly for three weeks.


# Pancreas Problems

The pancreas has two functions, to produce insulin and to produce digestive enzymes which are essential for the digestion of food.

## Acute Pancreatitis

If the pancreas becomes damaged or inflamed its cells can break apart releasing the digestive enzymes they contain. Unfortunately this can lead to the pancreas to start digesting itself with sometimes fatal results and as you can imagine this is a very painful condition. In a lot of cases the causes are not known. Clinical signs can be acute debilitating pain, cat may adopt a praying position to minimize the pain, there is vomiting, the cat may pass loose faeces yellow due to fat content, there may be undigested food in the faeces , shock, pale gums, rapid weak pulse, cat reluctant to move.

## Treatment

Best to see the vet here as you need fast acting drugs to ease the inflammation and pain.

The cat would probably have to be put on a special diet for a while depending on how extensive the damage is and may have to be supplemented with digestive enzymes

## Herbal Treatment

Here it would be best to use Homoeopathic treatment as this by passes the digestive system. This is a hard one to treat and would be best to start with a fast and see what happens from there, look at the herbal treatment for the chronic condition.

## Homoeopathic Treatment.

**Iris Vers** - This is a most important pancreatic remedy, stools are watery and light coloured or sometimes greenish, abdominal pain is severe. suggested potency is 6C giving one dose three times daily followed by 30C three times weekly for four weeks.

**Iodum 30C** - Stools are consistently frothy and fatty, suitable for the lean animal which has a voracious appetite and dry coat. Give one dose daily for two weeks.

**Pancreas 30C -** The pancreas nosode is of use along with the selected remedy. Give one dose daily for seven days.

# Chronic Pancreatitis

Not a dramatic condition but a slow decline in the functions of the pancreas with maybe a few mild acute episodes. The pancreas gradually produces less and less until there is not sufficient enzymes for digestion.

## Signs and Symptoms

The appetite is usually maintained and in many instances becomes excessive despite this there can be weight loss. Other symptoms are excessive thirst, ill formed bowel motions - greasy yellowish and may become rancid and foul smelling, undigested food in the faeces.

## Herbal Treatment

Pancreatic Enzymes can be supplemented and mixed with the cats food. Select herbs for the digestive system like bitters and cholagogues and anti inflammatories so as to help with the inflammation also demulcents may be of some use in soothing the irritated areas. Look at the diet to try and find the cause.

## Homoeopathic treatment

**Idum 30C** - This remedy is associated with voracious appetite and a inability to gain weight. It is well adapted to lean animals with dry harsh coats. Stools are frothy and contain fat globules. Lymphatic glands are often hard and smaller than usual. Give one dose daily for fourteen days.

# Diabetes

There are two types

## Diabetes Insipidus

This condition sometimes affects the older cat especially neutered males. The insulin secreting portion of the pancreas becomes deficient not making enough insulin that is required for the body. In this form the cat's kidneys are unable to concentrate the bodies waste products into a relatively small volume of urine especially as they now have to remove all this excess sugar from the blood stream. As a result the cat produces vast quantities of weak urine. Wasting is a common sequel in established cases and occasionally the animal will develop cataracts.

**Symptoms** - Can be increased thirst, increased volume of urine passed and increased frequency in urination.

## Treatment

It is hard to think of what to do here but the place to start should be the diet in which you would have to experiment to see what improves the condition. A Homoeopathic remedy you could try is

**Iris Vers** - This is a most important pancreatic remedy, stools are watery and light coloured or sometimes greenish, abdominal pain is severe. Suggested potency is 6C giving one dose three times daily followed by 30C three times weekly for four weeks.

**Diet** - Change the diet to a high protein one because protein is converted more slowly into glucose thus keeping the blood sugar stable.

### Diabetes Mellitus

This condition is similar to the human condition; the pancreas fails to produce enough insulin. Insulin is essential for the cells to utilize glucose and to enable glucose to enter the cell. Lack of insulin stops the supply of energy to the cells and overloads the bloodstream with sugar which forces the kidneys to start releasing the sugar in the urine.

**Symptoms** - Can be increased urine output, frequency of urination, thirst, hunger, weight loss.

Diagnoses are through blood sugar tests and urine test.

### Treatment

Treatment is insulin replacement like what is done in humans.

# Herbal Overview of the Digestive System

Unfortunately one of the main ways of diagnosing what sort of disease a animal has is to do a autopsy straight after it has died, this has to be done especially in fast acting diseases that kill fast. Always isolate the animal from the others and clean and disinfect where the animal has been so as to minimize the spread of infection. In dealing with problems of the digestive system its always best to start with a purge so as to clean the system and bowels out. This is very important especially when you do not know what you are dealing with because you are purging out hopefully most of the toxins that are causing the condition. After the purge isolate and fast the animal for 24 hours and see what happens. Always start on the Garlic and Echinacea straight away as the Echinacea is also used to treat septicemia and to attack blood borne toxins and with Garlic being antiviral and antibacterial we have together a good strong initial attack. If you look at the herbal treatment sections above you will see they cover most of the conditions of the digestive system and should give you helpful information. Below is a list of Herbal Actions that are used for the digestive system read through them and become familiar with them for in Herbal Medicine you always think in actions needed not the Herb needed this way the mind stays on the big picture.

# Herbal Actions for the Digestive System

**Anti-biotic** - Always start with Garlic as this is both anti-bacterial and anti-viral as well as being used for killing parasites and worms, your initial attack begins here.

**Herbs** - Echinacea, Garlic, Myrrh, Pau D' Arco, Reshi.

**Anti-emetic** - Can reduce a feeling of nausea and can help to relieve or prevent vomiting.

**Herbs** - Cayenne, Fennel, Meadowsweet, Peppermint.

**Anti-inflammatory** - Helps the body to combat inflammations, there will always be pain, heat and maybe fever when these are called for.  Herbs mentioned under demulcents will often act in this way especially when they are applied to coat for example a inflamed intestine or any other inflamed organ.(Slippery Elm).

**Herbs** - Cranesbill, Chamomile, Eyebright, Fennel, Feverfew, Ginger, Golden Rod, Ladys Mantle, Liquorice, Marshmallow, Meadowsweet, Marigold,  Pau D' Arco, Witch Hazel, Wormwood.

**Anti-microbial** - Helps the body destroy or resist pathogenic micro-organisms.

**Herbs** - Aniseed, Cayenne, Echinacea, Garlic, Gentian, Marigold, Myrrh, Peppermint, Rosemary, Rue, Sage, Thyme, Wormwood.

**Antispasmodic** - Prevents or eases spasms and cramps especially of the intestines.

**Herbs** - Aniseed, Angelica, Chamomile, Fennel, Rosemary, Rue, Sage, Skullcap, St John's Wort, Thyme, Valerian, Vervain.

**Anti-viral** - Astragalus, Cats claw, Echinacea, Garlic, Myrrh?, Shitake, St John's Wort, Pau D'Arco.

**Anthelmintic** - Destroys or expels worms from the digestive system.

**Herbs** - Garlic, Tansy, Wormwood, Thyme, Rue.

**Aperient** - Mild laxative.

**Herbs** - Burdock, Dandelion.

**Astringent** - Contracts  tissue which in turn reduces discharges, these herbs contain tannins. In the digestive system they can be used to stop diarrhoea and in the treatment of ulcers. Most astringents also have a anti-bacterial action.

**Herbs** - Agrimony, Bear Berry, Cranesbill, Comfrey, Eyebright, Golden Rod, Hops, Ladys Mantle, Marigold, Marshmallow, Meadowsweet, Nettles, Raspberry, Sage, Rosemary, Slippery Elm, Shepherds Purse, St John's Wort, Slippery Elm, Thyme, Witch Hazel, Yarrow.

**Bitters** - Herbs that taste bitter act as stimulating tonics for the digestive system.

**Herbs** -Burdock, Feverfew, Gentian, Hops, Horehound, Rue, Tansy, Wormwood.

**Carminative** - Stimulates peristalsis of the digestive system and relaxes the stomach and helps remove gas and wind from the system. These herbs are usually rich in volatile oils.

**Herbs** - Aniseed, Angelica, Cayenne, Chamomile, Fennel, Garlic, Ginger, Golden Rod, Hyssop, Horseradish, Juniper, Parsley, Peppermint, Penny Royal, Sage, Rosemary, Tansy, Thyme, Valerian, Wormwood.

**Cholagogue** - Stimulates the release of bile from the gallbladder which can relieve gallbladder problems, bile is also the body's natural laxative so cholagogues have a laxative effect as well.

**Herbs** - Agrimony, Blue Flag, Dandelion, Fumitory, Gentian, Marigold, Milk Thistle, Yellow Dock.

**Demulcent** - Soothes and protects irritated or inflamed internal tissues.

**Herbs** - Bear Berry, Corn Silk, Coltsfoot, Comfrey, Fenugreek, Liquorice, Marshmallow, Milk Thistle, Mullein, Oats, Plantain, Slippery Elm.

**Diaphoretic** - Aids the skin in the elimination of toxins and produces sweat thus reducing the temperature of fevers.

**Herbs** - Angelica, Black Cohosh, Cayenne, Chamomile, Elder, Elecampane, Fennel, Garlic, Ginger, Golden Rod, Guaiacum, Hyssop, Lime Blossom, Peppermint, Sarsaparilla, Thyme, Vervain, Yarrow.

**Hepatic** - Tones and strengthens the liver, may increase the flow of bile.

**Herbs** - Agrimony, Blue Flag, Dandelion, Fennel, Fumitory, Gentian, Horseradish, Hyssop, Motherwort, Milk Thistle, Vervain, Wormwood, Yarrow.

**Laxative** - Promotes the evacuation of the bowels.

**Herbs** - Burdock, Dandelion., Fumitory, Horseradish, Liquorice.

**Parasiticide** - Kills parasites and insects.

**Herbs** - Aniseed, Rosemary.

**Sialagogue** - Stimulates the secretion of saliva.

**Herbs** - Blue flag, Cayenne, Gentian, Ginger.

# Diseases of the Urinary System

## The Kidneys

The kidneys filter and remove toxic waste products from the cats blood via the urine. If the kidneys are not functioning properly waste products accumulate in the blood and have a toxic or poisoning effect on the cat. They also regulate calcium and Vitamin D levels, maintain the cat's level of hydration and secrete the hormone responsible for red blood cell production.

1. **Acute kidney problems** or infections don't happen often in cats but the symptoms are sudden onset, there may be depression and lack of appetite, temperature rise is common in the early stages, there is tenderness in the lumber area and arching of the back is seen, vomiting (may be blood tinged), thirst, inflammation of the mouth (often with difficulty swallowing), severe dullness, a decrease in urination, convulsions and coma. Causes can be bacterial or viral infections, toxins such as anti-freeze, herbicides and rat poisons.

2. **Chronic Kidney** disease occurs as the kidneys deteriorate slowly over a cat's lifetime. Especially common in cats over 9 years old. This is a common situation and is called Chronic Renal Disease. Old cats frequently show signs starting with great thirst, increased urinary output, loss of weight and condition. In more advanced cases you find uraemia (retention of waste products in the blood), vomiting, bad breath, a sore ulcerated mouth, anaemia, dehydration. In terminal cases death is preceded by vomiting of blood, convulsions and coma.

**Diet** - We used to advise a low protein diet as urea is a waste product of proteins and a sick kidney will have a hard time trying to get rid of this, but now they say this is not such a good idea and we should instead try to focus on keeping the phosphorus down instead. You can do this be replacing beef with chicken and turkey which are low in phosphorus, also try to keep the salt down. Give your cat a good quality low protein (eggs) high carbohydrate diet, glucose, honey and sugar are useful.

## Treatment for Kidney Problems

Fluid replacement is very important so always keep the cats water dish fill and handy. You can assess your cats state of dehydration by pinching the cats skin on the top of the neck for 5 seconds and then seeing how long it takes to flatten. The skin should pop back in 1 to 3 seconds if it does not the cat needs to be rehydrated. Most cats with kidney failure are also anaemic and will need B vitamins and iron.

## Herbal Treatment for the Acute Condition

As for any infections think of Echinacea and Myrrh and doses of Vitamin C. Other herbs for this condition to consider are Bearberry, Buchu and Corn Silk which are all urinary antiseptics and two of these herbs are demulcents so they would sooth the inflamed area. Other herbs that could be helpful are Angelica, Cleavers, Damiana, Golden Rod and Shepherds Purse.

## Homoeopathic Treatment of the Acute Condition

**Aconitum 30C** - This should be given in the early stages, at this stage the animal shows anxiety and distress and possibly even fear. This remedy will do much to relieve the patient of these anxieties and help calm them and sometimes it prevents the disease process going any further.

**Apis Mel 200C** - This is a most valuable remedy especially for the oedema and swelling it may also help with the pain, the animal is thirstless and shows a aversion to heat. It helps promote urination and will bring about a feeling of wellbeing.

**Arsen Alb 1M** - For animals which show dehydration and a harsh dry coat and have a thirst for small quantities of water often, the mucous membranes of the eyes are red and there may be vomiting and diarrhea. Symptoms are usually worse towards midnight when the patient becomes increasingly restless.

**Belladonna 200C** - The cat will exhibit signs of nervous system disturbance. The animal feels extremely hot with dilated pupils and a full bounding pulse, there are frequent attempts to pass urine which is scanty in amount and sometimes reddish brown in colour. Signs of nervous system involvement may be present such as excitability and possibly a tendency to convulsions.

**Phosphorus 200C** - An important remedy which will help to control vomiting which arises when liquids are rejected soon after ingestion. There may be a accompanying gingivitis with small haemorrhages present when this remedy is indicated.

**Urtica Urens 6X** - This remedy helps elimination of waste products via the urine and promotes urination. Another leading sign for this remedy is a rash on the skin.

## Herbal Treatment for the Chronic Condition

You really need to know the cause to be able to give the best treatment but if in doubt you can use all the herbs mentioned in the acute condition. For this condition I would be inclined to make up a tonic formula using the urinary anti septics so as to keep infections at bay along with the demulcents so as to sooth the effected areas and to this I would add Gravel root in case a stone is causing the problem and herbs like Chaparral, Cleavers and Damiana which are alterative and clean out the area. If diuretics are needed Dandelion leaf would be the best one to give.

## Homoeopathic Treatment for the Chronic Condition

**Arsen. Alb 30C** - The remedy to be considered when the patient shows excessive dehydration with increased thirst and dry coat. Itching of various areas may be pronounced and all symptoms are generally worse towards midnight, there is great restlessness. Give one dose three times daily for 10 days.

**Colchicum 30C** - There is increased urination with frequency. The urine can vary from clear to dark brown. There are usually accompanying joint pains indicated by stiffness and a inclination not to move. Abdominal flatulence may be more extreme and oedema may be present. Give one dose 3 times daily for 14 days.

**Phosphuros 30C** - This remedy has a beneficial tonic effect on the kidney parenchyma. Output of urine is increased and vomiting of stomach contents when they become warm is a strong guiding symptom for its use, small haemorrhages may appear on the gums. Give one dose twice daily for seven days. This remedy is probably one of the best to be considered

**Natrum Mur 200C**- Excessive urination and frequency is a notable feature when this remedy may be needed and this is often worse during the night. Mouth lesions in the form of superficial ulcers and blisters are often present while hawking and scraping of throat occurs. One dose 3 times weekly for 4 weeks.

## Urinary Tract Problems

Urine from the kidneys pass down tubes called ureters to the bladder where it is stored until being voided via the urethra. Feline lower urinary tract diseases called FLUTD, are common in cats affecting the bladder (cystitis) and the urethra (urethritis).

## Stones and Sand

Another problem that can happen are blockages somewhere down the line from little stones or sand which block off the line and cause a back log of urine. Symptoms can look like this - the cat will crouch uncomfortably over the litter and will strain to pass a little urine, the abdomen may become distended (do not squeeze tummy as the bladder may burst), the cat will probably become anxious and distressed. Blood may be passed in the urine.

Causes can be from being de-sexed to early, low fluid intake, too much dry food, old age, being overweight and lack of exercise. Stones which are mostly made up of phosphates usually have their origin in alkaline urine which can predispose the cat to urinary infections, these stones are the most common.

**Herbal Treatment -** the cat must have access to lots of fresh water, change the diet. The three different types of herbs we have to use here are the urinary antiseptics, the demulcents (so as to sooth raw areas) and the anti lithics. Don't forget to use our immune boosters if infection is present they are Echinacea, Garlic and Myrrh. Some good urinary antiseptics are Angelica, Bearberry and Buchu. Good demulcents for this system are Corn silk, Marshmallow and Bearberry. Some anti lithics are Cleavers, Bearberry and Gravel Root. Vegetables such as lovage, celery, asparagus and artichoke are good preventatives for stone formation and can be added to the diet in small quantities at first to see if they agree. Make sure the cat has lots of fresh water and drinks often. If the cat is drinking boar water stop this as it could be part of the cause.

## Homoeopathic Treatment

**Lycopodium 12C** - This remedy has a tonic action on the liver and will help to control the metabolism of that gland as a disturbed liver is frequently the cause of gravel formation. Subjects are thin and wizened looking showing reddish sediment in the urine. Give one dose twice daily for 21 days.

**Urtica Urens 6X** - Thickens the urine and removes the tendency to gravel formation by removing the basic salts that help form it, it will also increase the quantity of urine passed, there may be a skin rash, give one dose 3 times daily for 10 days.

**Calc Phos 30C** - A good constitutional remedy which will help regulate the calcium and phosphate metabolism and so prevent the formation of phosphates, it should be given as a routine remedy in young animals up till the age of one. One dose weekly for 8 weeks.

**Mag Mur 6C** - May help in preventing some forms of stones and may be given as a routine remedy if the urine shows suspicious deposits and there are other signs of stone formation.

# Cystitis

Cystitis is usually caused by a infection usually of a bacterial nature with the main culprits being E. Coli and Proteus which can be provoked by the cat holding on to its urine so access to its litter is important, the cat may also be fussy and not like using dirty litter.

## Signs and Symptoms

Squatting frequently to urinate, may frequently lick its genital area, urine may have blood in it or may smell stronger than usual ,may strain to urinate, the cat may cry out in pain, there is a temperature rise in the early stages. Treatment is usually antibiotics. It is best to deal with cystitis immediately as sometimes the infection can travel up the ureters and infect the kidneys.

## Herbal Treatment

The main herbs we use in cystitis are the urinary antiseptics with the best ones being Bearberry and Buchu. Cranberry juice is a good urinary antiseptic to. To the antiseptics we add demulcents which sooth the irritated tissues with the best one for this condition being Corn Silk. You could add to the formula Gravel Root if you think the cause of the condition could be from urinary stones or gravel. Other herbs to consider are Angelica, Yarrow, Agrimony, Cleavers, Damiana, Golden Rod, Juniper, Plantain and Shepherds Purse.

## Homoeopathic Treatment

**Aconitum 12X -** Will be of value in the early feverish phase of the acute stage, helping to calm the patient and allay pain and fear.

**Cantharis 6C -** One of the principle remedies employed, the patient strains violently and passes blood stained urine drop by drop with great frequency.

**Causticum 30C -** A useful remedy in the recurrent or chronic form and is especially adapted to the older animal. Follows well after Cantharis which may be needed if acute symptoms flare up in the chronic form.

# Herbal Overview of the Urinary System

Most infections get to the kidneys via the blood for the kidneys are the main filter of the blood removing wastes and water. Other infections can start off as cystitis and travel up the ureter and infect the kidney that way so you must always consider both ways. Always ask your self is the infection traveling from the kidney down or the bladder up? If you think it is the kidney put a leash on the animal and walk them in tight circles one way and then the other. If the animal complains it is probably the kidney. Urinary antiseptics are good for this system whether for treating infection or preventing it as in cases of stones scraping the sides as they go down leaving a wound ripe for infection. Also think of Cranberry for this system as it coats the pipes and stops bacteria getting a foot hold literally.

# Herbal Actions for the Urinary System

**Anti-biotic -** Chaparral, Echinacea, Garlic, Myrrh, Pau D' Arco.

**Anti-inflammatory -** Helps the body to combat inflammations.

**Herbs -** Cats Claw, Chaparral , Cleavers, Cranesbill, Eyebright, Ginger, Golden Rod, Guaiacum, Liquorice, Marshmallow, Pau D' Arco.

**Anti-lithic** - Prevent the formation of stones or gravel in the urinary system and helps the body to remove them.

**Herbs** - Bearberry, Corn Silk, Chaparral, Gravel Root, Horsetail.

**Anti-microbial** - Helps the body destroy or resist pathogenic micro-organisms.

**Herbs** - Echinacea, Garlic, Juniper, Myrrh,

**Astringent** - Contracts tissue which in turn reduces discharges, these herbs contain tannins.

**Herbs** - Agrimony, Cranesbill, Chaparral, Golden Rod, Horsetail, Shepherds Purse.

**Cystitis** - Agrimony, Bearberry, Buchu, Celery Seed, Corn Silk, Gravel Root, Golden Rod, Horsetail, Plantain,

**Demulcent** - Soothes and protects irritated or inflamed internal tissues.

**Herbs** - Bearberry, Corn Silk, Liquorice, Marshmallow, Plantain, Slippery Elm.

**Diuretic** - Increases the secretion and elimination of urine. Generally has a action on the kidneys.

**Herbs -** Agrimony Angelica, Bear Berry, Blue Flag, Burdock, Buchu, Broom, Coltsfoot, Chaparral, Corn Silk,  Dandelion Leaves, Elder, Fumitory, Golden Rod, Guaiacum, Gravel Root, Hawthorn, Horseradish, Horsetail, Juniper, Lime Blossom, Nettles, Pau D' Arco, Penny Royal, Plantain, Parsley,  Shepherds Purse, Sarsaparilla, Yarrow.

**Urinary Antiseptics** - These herbs have a antiseptic action as they pass through the system.

**Herbs** - Angelica, Bearberry, Buchu, Corn Silk, Golden Rod, Shepherds Purse, Yarrow.

# Nervous System Problems

## Signs and Symptoms

## Stagger Gait

If your cat staggers wobbles or falls over or generally has trouble standing upright this may be due to a disorder of the nervous system or a ear problem effecting balance.

Thing to look for

1.  Has the cat ingested poison?
2.  Are there signs of disease - vomiting, diarrhoea, dilated pupils etc.
3.  Has the cat been in a accident and hurt its back or could it be in shock.

## Trembling

Things to look for

1.  Has the cat been in a accident - Shock?
2.  Has the cat ingested poison.
3.  Are there signs of disease - vomiting, diarrhoea, dilated pupils etc.
4.  Are there any parasite dropping in the fur or are there any ticks.

## Paralysis

Thing to look for

1.  Any indications of a accident if so it may be a spinal injury.
2.  Does the paralysis affect only the back limbs if so this may indicate spinal disease or damage.
3.  Are the cats pupils dilated if so it may have encephalitis?
4.  Has the cat ingested poison?
5.  Are there any ticks on the cat.

**Poisons that cause nerve damage are** anti-freeze, aspirin, benzoic acid, insecticides, lead, mercury, metaldehyde (snail bait) and organophosphates (snail bait and other pesticides)

# Disease Conditions of the Nervous System

## Epilepsy

This is a disturbance in the functioning of the brain. The causes are often obscure but may be a tumour or injury. Symptoms are of fits, the cat keels over suddenly with little warning, frothing at the mouth, chattering its jaws and paddling frantically with its paws oblivious to its surroundings. After several minutes the animal will quieten lying still as if exhausted and then shortly get to its feet as it nothing has happened. Don't put your finger in the cats mouth as cats virtually never swallow there tongue. An investigation will have to be made to find the cause starting with a deficiency of Thiamine for this has been shown to cause fits when left out of the diet.

## Herbal Treatment

You need to try to prescribe on the whole picture of the cat and it may be worthwhile adding oats to the diet as this is a good nerve food. Herbs that have been used for epilepsy are Skullcap, Mistletoe, Gotu Kola, Hyssop and Passion Flower. To build up the nervous system and strengthen it think of Oats, Chamomile and Valerian.

## Homoeopathic Treatment

The following remedies may be found useful in controlling the condition though it will be found that some animals are resistant to treatment.

**Belladonna 30C -** This is one of the most frequently indicated remedies, for attacks associated with dilated pupils and throbbing pulse, the animal will usually feel abnormally hot and there is unconsciousness.

**Stramonium 30C** - This remedy is somewhat similar to the last one but there are usually signs before the fit such as staggering with a tendency to fall toward the left side, eyes are again dilated and staring. Dose once daily for 7 days.

**Cocculus 6C -** For long term cases and fits which come on associated with travel or unusual movement. The main use for this remedy lies more in the preventative sphere and is useful to ward off subsequent attacks. It should be given at regular intervals over a period of a few months.

**Ignatia 6C** - Consciousness is usually lost when this remedy is indicated. The head may be shaken to and fro and this precedes hysterical turns.

**Cuprum Met 6C** - A useful remedy when convulsions are associated more with meningitis then with encephalitis. The head usually assumes a lowered posture and there may be attempts to press it against any suitable object. Other signs for this remedy can be cramping and restricted movements. Dose 3 times daily for 14 days.

# Strokes

This sometimes appears in older cats and probably has its origins in a thrombosis which is a clot blocking a artery.

## Signs and Symptoms

After the initial onset that is usually sudden various degrees of immobility may arise e.g paralysis of the facial or head muscles or more extensive paralysis of one side of the body. Mild cases may show little more than incoordination and a tendency to circle one side or another. Disturbances of vision may be present as a cross - eyed appearance or maybe a discrepancy in pupil sizes. Involvement of lip muscles may lead to salivation and drooling.

## Herbal Treatment

Hardening of the arteries is probably the main cause for strokes so we will use our herbs that we use for this condition to attack the cause. The main herb is Hawthorn which we will use as solvent to the plaque, other herbs to add to this are Garlic (lowers Cholesterol), Linden Flower all so known as Lime flowers and works well with Hawthorn. Another herb to look at is Ginko Biloba. Brahmi a Indian herb is the specific for strokes in humans, it doesn't cure the damage done to the brain but help the brain rewire around the damaged area. In a human let's say the stroke paralysed one arm then what we do is tie the good arm to the waist, this forces the brain to rewire to get the bad arm going again though it takes time.

## Homoeopathic Treatment

**Aconitum 10 m** - The usually sudden onset calls for this remedy initially as it will quickly allay shock and enable other remedies to act better. The highest potency you have got should be given and repeated in 30 minutes time.

**Conium 30C** - Has a useful action in the older animal with one of its main symptoms being weakness in the hind legs or weakness of different kinds in the hind legs ranging from unsteady gait to a inability to rise with a progressive upwards paralysis.1 dose daily for 10 days.

**Arnica 200C -** Use this for the suddenness of the condition and as it is a injury involving blood vessels Arnica will help here. It is also said that over a period of time Arnica can dissolve clots.

Take one dose daily for 3 days.


# Myelitis and Spinal Cord Damage

Usually happens as a result of a accident. Myelitis is inflammation of the spinal cord and can be caused by bacteria spreading from infected tissues nearby (often a septic bite wound in the back). Other causes can be Viruses (rabies), parasites or poisons. Signs depend on which part of the spinal cord is affected and can include paralysis and back pain. Professional help is needed and an x-ray will probably need to be taken.

## Signs and Symptoms

Both motor and sensory nerve tracts may be involved giving rise to a variety of symptoms such as loss of sensation in the limbs and tail or paraplegia in those animals which are severely affected. A change of gait is not uncommon. There may be a loss of control over bladder and bowel functions.

## Herbal Treatment

Read what is written in this section for Encephalitis and Meningitis. Homoeopathy is the better action as it is faster acting. A good herb to check out is Hypericum also known as St John's Wort.

## Homoeopathic Treatment

**Conium Mac 30C -** This remedy is almost specific for those cases which show hind leg weakness ranging from slight ataxia to paraplegia where there is progressive upwards involvement of the disease process.

**Gelsemium 30C** - Mild cases showing a general weakness of the neuromuscular system may benefit from this remedy. Smaller peripheral nerves are very often affected more than the large nerve trunks e.g the nerves governing the throat and larynx, lassitude is a common feature.

**Causticum 30C** - A useful remedy for the older subject showing involvement of one particular nerve e.g the sciatic or radial giving rise to a localized paralysis. The subject may display sessile warts.

**Silicea 30C** - This remedy has a certain reputation in the treatment of spinal conditions and is worth considering if other symptoms agree, it is particularly indicated in the treatment of the lean or apparently less well-nourished animal.

# Encephalitis

This is inflammation of the brain itself and can be caused by septicaemia, bacteria spreading from a middle ear infection, viruses such as rabies and a few other causes.

## Signs and Symptoms

Symptoms can be variable and include dullness, fever, dilated pupils, staggering gait, paralysis, epilepsy and coma. Varying degrees of nervous excitement are at first seen in mild cases leading in more severe cases to convulsions. The eyes are usually staring and have a anxious or wild expression. The conjunctivae are red, facial twitching and head shaking may be present, the animal may cry out in pain, there is a staggering gait with stumbling and a tendency to fall forwards or backwards. This is a life threatening disease that needs immediate attention

## Herbal Treatment

Herbal treatment could be to slow for a fast acting disease as this but consider Garlic,Echinacea and Myrrh for bacterial and viral infections. Another herb to look at is St John's Wort because it is a Nervine anti-viral. Essential oils can cross the blood brain barrier and could be a fast way of getting into the area so try maybe Garlic oil ,Lavender oil, Myrrh, Thyme or Eucalyptus diluted and rubbed in the area as these are all anti microbials. I have not heard of essential oils being used for this condition but as a last desperate resort I would try it. Homoeopathy is the better action to take as it is faster acting then herbal medicine.

## Homoeopathic Treatment

**Aconitum 30C** - If attacks come on suddenly this remedy will help allay shock and limit the scope of the attack.

**Belladonna 30C** - This is one of the chief remedies for relieving convulsions in the acute stage. Indications for its use are dilated pupils, throbbing pulse and redness of eyes.

**Stramonium 30C** - This remedy may be useful for the less acute case which shows a staggering gait with a tendency to fall towards the left side or even backwards. Abdominal symptoms such as colic and diarrhoea may accompany these attacks. Convulsive movements of the head are present and sight is usually lost.

**Conium Mac 30C** - Useful in the older animal, weakness of different kinds in the hind legs ranging from unsteady gait to a inability to rise with a progressive upwards paralysis

# Herbal Overview of the Nervous System

One of the most important herbs in this system is Hypericum also known as St John's Wort. This herb is anti-viral, antibacterial, anti-inflammatory, a sedative and one of our main first aid remedies for wounds which helps relieve pain and can kill the tetanus bacteria and this is only mentioning a part of its uses, always consider this when there are problems with this system especially if you don't know what the problem is. Another good herb for rebuilding this system is Oats which is a Nervine tonic also think of Valerian which is our main Tranquilliser but also a good tonic for this system. A lot of the herbs mentioned below are used in a lot of other body systems as well so when you want the action of a Nervine to use in another system try to match the herb to one used in that system as well.

# Herbal Actions for the Nervous System

**Antispasmodic** - Prevents or eases spasms and cramps.

**Herbs** - Aniseed, Angelica, Black Cohosh, Chamomile, Fennel, Horehound, Hyssop, Lime Blossom, Mistletoe, Motherwort,

Rosemary, Rue, Sage, Skullcap, St John's Wort, Thyme, Valerian, Vervain.

**Analgesic -** Herbs that reduce pain.

**Herbs** - Chamomile, Dong Quai, Hops, Ladys Mantle, Passion Flower, St John's Wort, Skullcap, Valerian, Wild Yam, Withania.

**Anti-depressive** - Damiana, Rosemary, Skullcap, St John's Wort, Valerian, Vervain.

**Hypnotic** - This means helps you to go asleep.

**Herbs** - Chamomile, Hops, Passion Flower, Valerian.

**Nervine** - Has a beneficial effect on the nervous system, acts like a tonic to this system.

**Herbs** - Black Cohosh, Chamomile, Hops, Lime Blossoms, Mistletoe, Motherwort, Oats, Peppermint, Rosemary, Skullcap, St John's Wort, Tansy, Thyme, Valerian, Vervain, Wormwood.

**Sedative** - Calms the nervous system and reduces stress and nervousness throughout the body.

**Herbs** - Black Cohosh, Chamomile, Hops, Hyssop, Motherwort, Skullcap, St John's Wort, Valerian , Vervain.

# Disease Conditions and Injuries of the Bones and Muscles

## Signs and Symptoms

Most of the main health problems here are due to fights and accidents. Diseases of this system are fairly rare in cats though arthritis can catch up to them in old age.

## Limping

Things to look for

1.  Does the cat seem in pain when you touch the affected limb, indicates injury or infection.
2.  Is a single limb affected, if so is it thicker than the other one, it may be fractured or sprained.
3  Is there any blood on the limb, the cat may have been in a accident.
4.  Is there a swelling on the limb, a tumour may be the cause.

## Swollen Legs and Feet.

A sudden swelling of the cat's legs or feet is most likely to be the result of an infection.

Things to look for

1.  Has your cat been in a fight, a bite may have caused an infection.
2.  Is a single limb affected, it may be fractured or have a tumour.
3.  Does the cat look pot-bellied, circulatory or kidney problems may of caused oedema.
4.  Does your pet seem stiff or have difficulty in moving around especially after a period of rest. It may have arthritis or another bone disease.

## Sprains

Sprains, strains and bruises consist of damage to the soft tissues surrounding and supporting the bones. Give your normal first aid treatment here starting with a cold pack. There is no fever with sprains so check as fever can be a sign of infection. A x-ray may be needed.

## Homoeopathic Treatment

**Arnica 6C**- For the shock and bruised sore pains. Arnica cream can also be applied as long as the skin is not broken.

**Bellis Perennis 6C** - Deeper acting then arnica, intense soreness of the muscles, where swellings and lumps remain after the injury.

**Ruta 6C** - If the bones inside or near the joint feel bruised

## Fractures

A complete break results in the inability of the limb to support weight and there may be some deformity in the limb. Usually there is a lot of swelling and shock. Use normal first aid procedures, support the limb or patient and transport for x-rays and further treatment.

## Common fractures are

Broken Jaws - from falling from heights, jump gone wrong.

Broken Tail - from getting jammed, crushed etc.

Broken Pelvis - Mostly from car accidents.

**Herbs** - Comfrey

## Homoeopathic Treatment

**Arnica 6C** - For the shock and bruised sore pains. Arnica cream can also be applied as long as the skin is not broken.

**Calc Phos 6X** - Helps in nutrition especially of the bones and promotes the knitting together of the bones. Help fractures heal much faster. Can be used in alternation with Symphytum.

**Symphytum 6C** - More commonly known as comfrey or knit bone or bone set. The name says it all. Promotes fast healing of bones, use with Calc Phos 6X. Take both 3 times daily till recovered.

# Dislocations

The signs of dislocation are similar to those of fracture but are usually milder. Dislocated bones are usually manipulated back into position under anaesthesia then the problem is to prevent the damaged and unstable joint from re dislocating. Sometimes the limb is bandaged in position other times surgery is needed.

**Herbs** - Comfrey

## Homoeopathic Treatment

**Arnica 6C** - For the shock and bruised sore pains. Arnica cream can also be applied as long as the skin is not broken.

**Bellis Perennis 6C** -  Deeper acting then arnica, intense soreness of the muscles, where swellings and lumps remain after the injury.

**Ruta 6C** - If the bones inside or near the joint feel bruised

# Myositis

Inflammation of muscle fibres leading to degeneration in prolonged cases. The cause may be systemic (Bacterial infection) or traumatic (injury).

## Signs and Symptoms

There may be swelling of the muscle involved but frequently no signs are evident except for the fact that the animal cries out on being moved or lifted. Various postures are assumed according to the muscles affected eg the arching of the back when the lumber muscles are affected or maybe a board like feeling on the abdomen which indicates pain of the muscles at that region.

## Herbal Treatment

If the cause is from bacterial infection then we would use our immune boosting herbs so as to start fighting the infection, these are Echinacea, Myrrh and Garlic. If inflammation is present treat with anti inflammatories especially the ones that are pain killers - St John's Wort and Devils Claw.  If the inflammation was caused by injury try some of the First Aid remedies such as a compress of Arnica Lotion. Don't forget to look at the Homoeopathic First Aid remedies.

## Homoeopathic Treatment

**Aconitum 30C** - Should always be considered in the early stages and will bring about relief from pain especially if the origin is bacterial. It will allay any tendency to shock if the condition arises quickly.

**Rhus Tox 6C** - Indicated  when the animal gains relief from movement even though the initial movement is painful, symptoms may be more on the left side of the body then the right, indicated when severe wetting or prolong dampness is associated with the onset of the symptoms. Dose is twice daily for 21 days.

**Bryonia 6C -** Movement is resented when Bryonia is indicated. The animal will seek to lie on the affected muscles and pressure on them gives ease, warmth is usually useful also. Dose twice daily for 15 days.

**Causticum 12C -** This remedy is associated with a accompanying contraction of tendons and a stiffness of muscles, warmth gives relief, more adaptable to the older patient with unsteadiness of gait. Dose is twice a day for 14 days.

**Gelsemium 12C -** Weakness and a tendency to paralysis is the keynote of this remedy. There may be generalised involvement of all muscles and the trouble is usually systemic in origin, an attempt to exercise the animal can lead to collapse and severe fatigue. Dose daily for 14 days.

# Osteoarthritis

Degenerative joint disease where the articular cartilages become eroded and bony exostoses occur at the margin of the joints. The hip and stifle joints are the ones most commonly affected.

All though age plays a part there can be other causes such as systemic or metabolic disturbances. Progressive mild inflammation in the joint over a period of time is more likely to produce osteoarthritis than any other predisposing factor. Osteoarthritis particularly affects the load bearing bones of the body. Being overweight adds to the wear and tear of the joints. Once the cartilage degenerates the cushioning effect is lost within the joint and the joint capsule now becomes involved and the situation becomes worse.

## Signs and Symptoms

Lameness is the main sign and it could involve several joints. An unwillingness to use the affected part results in muscular wasting of the area, later signs include thickening of the joint, the worst affected limb may be held in a flexed manner.

## Herbal Treatment

Nutrition wise for the early stages you can give Calcium, Vitamin D, Magnesium and Manganese so as to try to stop the condition from getting worse. Glucosamine and Chondroitin Sulphate can help stimulate the rebuilding of cartilage and help in the early stages of arthritis.

Arthritis with lots of pain and inflammation needs the use of the anti-inflammatory herbs, good ones to use for this condition are Devils Claw and St John's Wort as these act as good pain killers as well. Other herbs to use are the alteratives which clean out the area and the system some good ones are Burdock, Garlic, Sarsaparilla and Chaparral which has a antioxidant action as well. Diuretic herbs are also used for this condition as they help to remove the metabolic waste and toxins which usually result from the constant inflammation and help the kidneys flush this waste out, some good ones are Celery seed, Juniper (these two are best used together) and Dandelion leaf. Other herbs to look at for arthritis are Black cohosh, Cats Claw, Guaiacum, Nettles, Wild yam and Yellow dock. Add Liquorice to the formula at about 10% as this will help in the assimilation of the formula into the body.

## Homoeopathic Treatment

Not an easy condition to treat. Start treatment as early as possible so as to slow down deterioration. Useful remedies for the early inflammatory stages are.

**Rhus Tox 6C -** This remedy is indicated when the animal's symptoms are eased after a short period of movement, there may be initial stiffness on first moving.

**Bryonia 6C -** The indications for this remedy are the opposite of the above, the animal prefers to remain still and any movement causes distress and sometimes acute pain evidenced by the animal crying out.

**Caulophyllum 6C -** This remedy could be indicated if the condition is confined to the smaller joints eg, carpus, tarsus and the joints of the toes.

**Formic Acid 6X -** Stiffness in joints, right side mostly affected, pains worse motion, better pressure, weakness of lower extremities, stiff and contracted joints.

**Calc Flour 30C -** May be needed in the latter stages once the exostoses and joint swellings develop. The carpus is the main joint affected when this remedy is indicated. There may be accompanying cystic tumours around the joint.

# Arthritis due to Infection

This is caused by pyogenic bacteria getting in the joint mainly from injury the main organisms are Streptococci and Staphylococci .

## Signs and Symptoms

There is a initial temperature rise and febrile signs develop. The affected joint becomes swollen, tense and hot. Pain is obvious by the onset of severe lameness. Examination may reveal the presence of punctures on the skin and the appearance of a purulent exudate.

## Herbal Treatment

For this condition think of our infection fighting herbs such as Echinacea, Garlic and Myrrh.

If the skin is broken and you think the infection got in this way apply a lotion of Calendula and Hypericum (St John's Wort) to the area. To our infection fighting herbs you can add some of the anti-inflammatories, alteratives and diuretics that are mentioned in Osteo Arthritis. Add Liquorice to the formula at about 10% as this will help in the assimilation of the formula into the body.

## Homoeopathic Treatment

**Aconitum 30C -** This should be given as soon as possible in the early febrile stage.

**Ferrum Phos 6C -** This also is a good remedy for the initial feverish stage more often indicated when throat symptoms accompany the invasive process.

**Belladonna 30C -** Indicated when the patient presents a excitable picture with dilated pupils, throbbing arteries and a hot skin.

**Bryonia 6C -** Symptoms worse for movement, relief from pain on pressure over the joint and a possible involvement with the respiratory tract. The joint is usually extremely hard and tense.

**Apis Mel 6C -** If the synovial sheaf of the joint becomes oedematous indicated by swelling this remedy may help. The patient is made worse by heat in any form and does not drink much.

**Ledum 6C -** The remedy of choice if the arthritis has been caused by the penetration of a sharp object giving rise to a puncture wound.

**Iodum 6C** - This is a remedy which sometimes gives good results in the less acute case especially when the joint pains are worse at night. The patient is often thin with a voracious appetite and the skin is dry and withered looking.

**Rhus Tox 6C** - The indications for this remedy are relief from movement although there may be initial stiffness on rising. There may be accompanying skin symptoms of a vesicular itchy nature.

**Silica 30C** - This remedy is indicated in the more chronic case. There may be involvement of neighbouring lymphatic glands showing cold abscesses.

# Osteomyelitis

This term refers to a infection of the bone in the acute form which arises when pyogenic bacteria gain entrance to the medulla of the bone either through blood transfer or via compound fractures.

Cat's bones lie fairly close to the surface of the body and are in general less protected by the layers of soft tissue then humans or dogs. During a fight the sharp teeth of a feline adversary can easily penetrate to the bone therefore limb or tail bone infections are quite common. If the marrow is involved osteomyelitis may develop. Wounds must therefore be treated before any serious infection can take hold. Chronic osteomyelitis can develop when infections reach the periosteum and can follow puncture wounds and bites. The main pyogenic organisms associated with this disease are Staphylococci and to a lesser extent Streptococci.

## Herbal Treatment

For this condition think of our infection fighting herbs such as Echinacea, Garlic and Myrrh.

If the skin is broken and you think the infection got in this way apply a lotion of Calendula and Hypericum to the area. Treat the symptoms as you see them, if there is inflammation use the anti inflammatories, alteratives may be needed as well so as to clean out the area and system, some examples of herbs that have both of these actions are Devils Claw, Figwort and Sarsaparilla.

## Signs and Symptoms

Acute disease is characterised by lameness, febrile attacks and swelling of the limb. Sinus formation with purulent discharge is often the early sign of the chronic form and febrile signs are much less evident. X-ray is a good way for diagnosis.

## Homoeopathic Treatment

**Aconitum 30C** - Should always be given in the early febrile stage and may have to be repeated for one or two doses.

**Hepar Sulph 30C -** In the acute form accompanying severe pain this could prove a very useful remedy. A guiding symptom for its use is extremely sensitive to pain.

**Ruta 6c -** This remedy has a beneficial action on infections or inflammations of the periosteum and should be of good use in the acute form and may prevent the chronic from arising.

**Calc Phos 30C and Calc Carb 30C** - These two remedies could prove useful in treatment of the young animal that is still developing.

**Silica 30C** - A suitable remedy for the chronic form where sinuses have formed.

**Symphytum 200C -** This remedy should help allay the tendency to any weakening of bone structure and is generally a good healing agent.

# Osteoporosis

A condition in which bones become increasingly porous. It is due to metabolic upsets and may follow a systemic disease. Diagnosis depends on X -ray but symptoms can be an increased tendency to fractures. One cause is an all meat diet so check out nutrition.

## Herbal Treatment

This really depends on what is the cause of the problem is it nutrition, assimilation or is it a metabolic type of problem caused by a problem with the liver. I think here it is best to find the cause before using herbs.

## Homoeopathic Treatment

**Calc Phos 30C -** This is a very useful remedy for the younger animal in the growing stage as it exerts a profound influence on the development of bone and muscle. More suitable for lean animals.

**Calc Carb 30C -** This remedy has a action similar to the above one but it suits the fat animal more than the lean one.

**Calc Fluor 30C -** The fluoride of calcium is a good tissue remedy and is instrumental in hardening bone and strengthening the periosteum.. Dose daily for 21 days.

**Silicea 30C -** This is a good tissue remedy exerting a beneficial action on the skeletal in general.

## Herbal Overview of the Muscular Skeletal System

For bruising think about Arnica in a lotion and use the Homoeopathic dose internally, for broken bones think about Comfrey as its old name is knit bone. For arthritis and rheumatism use your Anti Rheumatics, Anti Inflammatorys and Analgesics but also think of Celery Seed as this is called the acid remover and another herb to think of is Meadowsweet as this herb is called the acid balancer. It is usually the high acid in the system that irritates the joints and starts the inflammation so these 2 herbs could remove the cause for the condition, also consider diet as a diet high in protein will create a lot of acid waste. For blood borne bacterial infections think of the Alteratives (blood cleansers) and Anti Bacterials especially our main ones Garlic and Echinacea. If there is damage to the joints use a nutritional supplement with these 3 together - Glucosamine Sulphate, Chondroitin and MSM as these together will help rebuild the joints.

## Herbal Actions for the Muscular Skeletal System

**Alterative -** Herbs that gradually restore proper function to the body, they increase health and vitality. They were once known as the blood cleansers.

**Herbs -** Black Cohosh, Blue Flag, Burdock, Chaparral, Echinacea, Garlic, Nettles, Pau D'Arco ,Sarsaparilla, Yellow Dock.

**Analgesic -** Herbs that reduce pain.

**Herbs** - Black Cohosh, Chamomile, Hops, Meadowsweet, Pau D'Arco, Peppermint, Skullcap, St John's Wort, Valerian.

**Anti-biotic** - Chaparral, Echinacea, Garlic, Myrrh, Pau D' Arco.

**Antispasmodic** - Prevents or eases spasms and cramps.

**Herbs** - Angelica, Black Cohosh, Chamomile, Skullcap, St John's Wort, Valerian.

**Anti-inflammatory -** Helps the body to combat inflammations.

**Herbs** - Cats Claw, Devils Claw, Chaparral , Feverfew, Ginger, Guaiacum, Liquorice, Meadowsweet, Pau D' Arco, Sarsaparilla, St John's Wort, Willow Bark.

**Anti-viral** - Astragalus, Cats claw, Echinacea, Garlic, Myrrh?, St John's Wort, Pau D'Arco.

**Anti-Rheumatic** - Angelica, Burdock, Black Cohosh, Chaparral, Cats Claw, Celery Seed, Dandelion, Garlic, Guaiacum, Nettles, Willow Bark, Yellow Dock.

**Rubefacient** - Causes a gentle local irritation to the skin which stimulates the capillaries to open increasing the blood flow.

**Herbs** - Cayenne, Garlic, Ginger, Horseradish, Nettles, Peppermint Oil, Rosemary Oil, Rue.

# Cardiovascular Problems

The circulatory system has two main functions, transporting oxygen and other vital materials around the body and combating infection. Unlike us cats aren't prone to heart disease and strokes, blood problems are the main threat to cats. Simple blood disorders such as anaemia are fairly common in cats. The normal heart rate for a cat is fast, 100 to 240 beats per minute. The cat's heart beat can be felt by placing your fingers on the left side of the chest just behind and above the elbow. With each heart beat a pulse can be felt in the major arteries the most convenient artery to feel for this is the femoral artery at the top of the hind legs.

## Heart Failure and Disease

As cats get older the heart valves may get weaker or become blocked, or the heart may just get tired, other causes can be a bacterial or viral infection that damages the heart muscle or the sack surrounding the heart.

## Signs of heart disease can include

1. A tendency to tire easily.
2. Breathlessness and heavy breathing.
3. A pale or bluish tinge to the gums.
4. Coughing especially early in the morning, wheezing, gasping and respiratory distress.
5. Exercise intolerance, tires easily, spends most of the day sleeping,
6. Restlessness, edgy, nervous, can't seem to get comfortable.

**Herbal Treatment** - Really depends on the cause. If the cause is a bacterial or viral infection then the herbs to look at would be Echinacea, Myrrh and Garlic. If the cause is from old age then the herb would be Hawthorn but whatever the cause always consider Hawthorn.

## Homoeopathic Treatment

**Adonis 4X -** This is one of the best remedies for valvular disease. Urine output is decreased and the urine contains albumen casts, the heart action is exaggerated, give one dose 3 times daily for 21 days.

**Convallaria 4X** - The pulse is full and intermittent, and the animal is disinclined to move, give 1 dose 3 times daily for 21 days.

**Lillium Tig 6C** - The pulse is small and rapid but weak when this remedy is indicated, even slight movement exacerbates the condition, sometimes acts better in the female, dose 3 times daily for 30 days.


# Stroke

**See Nervous System**


# Leukaemia

This is fairly common in cats and is caused by a virus; Feline leukaemia is contagious and is spread by direct contact. Some cats are naturally resistant to it while others develop immunity to it without showing to many signs and then there are the unlucky ones that get the disease. Once infected signs may be anaemia, weakness, loss of weight, vomiting, diarrhoea and respiratory problems.

Most of these animals are put down so as to control the disease.

Herbally  you could try the alteratives with the antivirals. See Chaparral.

# Anaemia

Is a reduction in the number of circulating red blood cells which causes a lack of oxygen, there are many reasons why this happens. The signs of anaemia are pale eye and mouth membranes, in advanced cases there are signs of oxygen hunger which are weakness, breathlessness, fatigue and restlessness.  Try to find the cause and treat the cause. The vet will diagnose by blood sample.

## Some reasons for anaemia.

1.   Parasites eg worms sucking blood.
2.   Poisons a good example is lead another is bacterial toxins from a infection.
3.   Loss of blood from a accident or internal bleeding somewhere.
4.   Some disease for example tumour of the bones, chronic kidney disease, TB.
5.   Poor diet especially if it's deficient in B complex or Iron.

## Signs and Symptoms

The rate of breathing may be increased along with the heart rate. There will be tiredness and weakness, mucous membranes will look pale, are the gums pale.

## Homoeopathic Treatment

**Arsen Alb 1M** - This deeply acting remedy will aid those cases showing extreme weakness and exhaustion with accompanying restlessness and thirst for small amounts of water. It has been used before with good results in the treatment of chronic Anaemia. 1 dose daily for 21 days.

**Merc Sol 6C** - Mercury produces severe anaemia and is a remedy which should be considered when its other symptoms are present e.g excess salivation and slimy diarrhoea and maybe skin eruptions. Dose 3 time daily for10 days.

**Silica 200C -** This is a remedy to consider if it is thought that the condition has arisen as a result of long standing infections especially if accompanied by general malnutrition, silica also has a specific action on bone disorders. Dose twice weekly for 8 weeks.

**Ferr Phos 6X -** Most health shops will have this in the Biochemic Cell Salts and it may give the cat a boost.

# The Female Reproductive System

## Acute Mastitis

### Inflammation of the Mammary

This condition is sometimes seen after parturition when one or more glands become swollen, hot and tender to touch, the milk becomes curdled and yellow after a while and in neglected cases discolouration of the mammary region occurs. The cat is obviously in pain and discomfort and has an anxious expression.

### Herbal Treatment

Humans sometimes use a cabbage leaf poultice for this condition, get some cabbage leafs and pound them so they are bruised all over and apply to the affected area, I'll leave you to figure out how to do this as I aren't all that sure myself as usually women use an oversized bra to hold the leaves in place . Photolacca (Poke Root) Tincture in very small doses is the main herb for mastitis though I believe the Homoeopathic potency is far better and faster acting then the tincture. After the Homoeopathic Dose you could make a lotion of Photolacca but make it a very mild lotion as this is a strong remedy so make it about 1 to 20 in strength. The main immune boosting herbs should also be used these are Echinacea, Garlic and Myrrh as well as the alteratives such as Cleavers.

### Homoeopathic Treatment

**Aconitum 12C -** Should be given in the early stages if possible. It will reduce anxiety and help calm the patient.

**Belladonna 200C -** Indicated when the glands are swollen, hot and tense, dilated pupils and a full and bounding pulse are present, increased sensitivity or excessive excitability may be seen.

**Apis Mel 30C -** Where oedema and stinging pain is present.

**Phytolacca 30C -** This is a valuable remedy as it has a selective action on the mammary gland. The inflammation may take the form of nodular patches of hard tissue while clots in the milk usually disappear under its influence.

**Bryonia 30C -** Useful remedy when the gland is excessively hard, there may be attendant constipation and respiratory upset such as pleurisy, general stiffness of limbs is present.

**Hepar Sulph 200C -** The cat exhibits aversion to touch indicating excessive tenderness and pain. Mammary secretion is probably thin and purulent.

# Acute Metritis

Metritis or inflammation of the womb can be acute or chronic. The acute condition is associated with the birth complex and runs a short course of up to five days. Chief among the causes of this condition is the retained placenta together with infection which gains entrance to the genital tract as a result of faulty obstetrical procedure.

## Signs and Symptoms

There is a rise in temperature and the cat is uneasy and lethargic. There may be diarrhea and vomiting along with signs of dehydration. The eyes are sunken and have a anxious expression. Thirst is increased but the appetite is poor or absent. Uterine discharges are present and vary in character from muco - purulent in mild cases to dark brown containing blood stained material in the more severe form.

## Herbal Treatment

We will start off by telling you how this problem on the pregnancy side could have probably been avoided in the first place. If the cat was given the herbs Raspberry or Squaw Vine in the last months of pregnancy these herbs would have toned and strengthened the uterus and the problem may of been avoided. At the onset of labour if the herb Golden Seal was used it could of given the cat the extra strength and energy to have a successful and problem free labour, this usually works by making the contractions stronger. When the kittens are born it is usually when they start to suckle that triggers the expulsion of the placenta. Inflammations of the uterus arising from infection should be treated with the main immune boosting herbs mainly Echinacea, Garlic and another good one if you have got it is Myrrh. To these herbs consider adding Lady's Mantle (astringent) Black or Blue Cohosh, or Saw Palmetto. Cleavers could be used as a Alterative for cleaning out the system. A lotion of Calendula could be used to clean the outside area especially if it is red and sore.

## Homoeopathic Treatment

Treatment should be started as bad signs start to appear after parturition especially after dead kittens and a difficult labour.

**Aconitum 30C -** Should be given at once so as to quickly allay shock, fear and anxiety and regulate the circulation.

**Belladonna 30C -** Indicated when the animal is hot to touch with a full bounding pulse and dilated pupils. Signs of cerebral excitement may be present with extreme cases convulsions.

**Apis Mel 30C -** Also useful in the early stages when a degree of oedema will be present in the uterine lining.

**Lillum Tig 30C -** A good general remedy for uterine congestion leading to blood stained discharges and straining in the pelvic region.

**Secale 6C -** Haemorrhages are present when this remedy is considered, the blood is fluid and dark, the patient is cadaverous looking with cold extremities which are deficient in blood supply.


# Herbal Overview of the Reproductive System

Herbs to think of when a miscarriage is suspected are False Unicorn Root, Lady's Slipper, Blue Cohosh, Black Haw, Wild Yam, and Cramp Bark. The main herbs to think of for pregnancy are Raspberry, Squaw Vine and Shepherds Purse. Below are some of the actions to consider for this system. In the Astringents the herbs underlined are the best to use to stop bleeding. Use the Alteratives for Chronic diseases of this system and maybe add some of the Emmenagogues to them after reading up on the individual herbs and adding the one that works in the direction you want.

# Herbal Actions for the Reproductive System

**Alterative** - Herbs that gradually restore proper function to the body, they increase health and vitality. They were once known as the blood cleansers.

**Herbs** - Black Cohosh, Dong Quai, Damiana, Skullcap.

**Anti-biotic** - Chaparral, Echinacea, Garlic, Myrrh, Pau D' Arco, Reshi.

**Anti-fungal** - Marigold, Cats Claw, Pau D' Arco, Myrrh, Sweet Violets.

**Anti-inflammatory** - Helps the body to combat inflammations. Herbs mentioned under demulcents, emollients and vulneraries will often act in this way especially when they are applied externally.

**Herbs** - Cranesbill, Chamomile, Eyebright, Feverfew, Ginger, Golden Rod, Lady's Mantle, Liquorice, Marshmallow, Meadowsweet, Marigold, Pau D' Arco, St John's Wort, Witch Hazel.

**Anti Tumor** - Burdock, Cleavers, Reshi, Shitake, Sweet Violets.

**Antispasmodic** - Prevents or eases spasms and cramps.

**Herbs** - Aniseed, Angelica, Black Cohosh, Chamomile, Fennel, Hyssop, Motherwort, Rosemary, Rue, Sage, Skullcap, St John's Wort, Thyme, Valerian, Vervain.

**Anti-viral** - Astragalus, Cats claw, Echinacea, Garlic, Myrrh?, Shitake, St John's Wort, Pau D'Arco.

**Astringent** - Contracts tissue which in turn reduces discharges, these herbs contain tannins.

**Herbs** - Agrimony, Cranesbill, Eyebright, Golden Rod, Lady's Mantle, Marigold, Raspberry, Shepherds Purse, St John's Wort, Witch Hazel.

**Emmenagogue** - Stimulates and normalizes the menstrual flow, tonics for the female reproductive system.

**Herbs** - Black Cohosh, Chamomile, Fenugreek, Gentian, Ginger, Juniper, Lady's Mantle, Marigold, Motherwort, Parsley, Penny Royal, Peppermint, Parsley, Raspberry, Sage, Rosemary, Rue, Shepherds Purse, St John's Wort, Tansy, Thyme, Valerian, Vervain, Wormwood, Yarrow.

**Galactagogue** - Helps increase the flow of milk in females.

**Herbs** - Aniseed, Fennel, Fenugreek, Milk Thistle, Raspberry, Vervain.

# Ears, Eyes and Teeth

## Otitis Media

This is inflammation of the middle ear and surrounding structures. The condition is frequently of bacterial origin and is often accompanied by nervous signs in a cat.

## Signs and Symptoms

Signs of this disorder include loss of hearing and a sense of balance. The cat may be staggering to one side or doing exaggerated limb movements. Moving in a circular pattern can develop along with the same kind of movement in the head.

## Herbal Treatment

Try to find the cause, is it a acute infection, tooth ache, from sinus problems etc. Recurring ear infections need professional help so as to build up the immune system to cope. For example a Professional may think of for a internal formula Anti microbials - Echinacea, Garlic and Lymphatics - Cleavers, Fenugreek with maybe Anti Catarrhals - Elder, Golden Rod along with Ginkgo to force the formula into the head. Seek medical help if the pain is excessive or there is pain in the mastoid bone (behind the ear) or any discharge. The juice of garlic or alternatively onion in olive oil warmed to body temperature but no more can be put in the ear but only if the drum is not perforated. If the drum is perforated they will be in great pain and there may be a discharge. To get the juice from a onion slice it thinly into circles and lay flat in a saucer and sprinkle a bit of sugar on it then put another layer of onion more sugar etc and keep building it up. When finished leave for at least a hour and the sugar will draw out the juice.

Ear drops - Garlic, Mullein and Hypericum (for pain), Onion poultice.

## Homoeopathic Treatment

**Aconitum 30C -** Should be given as the first remedy as soon as the problem is noted, especially if the condition came on fast.

**Stramonium 30C -** When there is a tendency for the animal to fall towards the left side, give daily for 10 days.

**Cicuta Virosa 30C -** Indicated for head symptoms such as bending the head backwards on the neck or showing a s shaped curve. Dose daily for 14 days.

**Agaricus 1M -** General incoordination of movement giving a drunk type of appearance, inability to stand properly and exaggerated limb movement. Dose daily for 10 days.

**Hepar Sulph 200C -** Extreme sensitivity to touch indicating pain. Dose daily for 5 days.

**Belladonna 200C -** When there is central nervous system involvement leading to fits, pupils may be dilated and there may be a bounding pulse. Dose 3 times weekly for 3 weeks.

# Eyes

## Cataract

A clouding of the lens of the eye that may affect one or both eyes making it difficult for the cat to see thing normally. Most cataracts get gradually worse. This can be a problem in the aged cat. Diabetes is also a common cause of cataracts in cats along with trauma injury to the eye.

### Signs and Symptoms

A slight greying of the eyes is the first noticeable symptom. Where they are hereditary they will start to appear when the cat is a kitten and progressively get worse till blind which is usually 2 to 3 years. As the condition worsens the cat will become more anxious in unfamiliar surroundings.

### Homoeopathic Treatment

**Calc Fluor 30C -** Give in the early stages so as to stop or prevent any further deterioration. Dose daily for 14 days.

**Silicea 200C -** This is the main remedy to consider in established cases and it may help the body to resorb the cataract. Give one dose twice weekly for 8 weeks.

**Nat Mur 30C** - For when the condition is accompanied by kidney involvement. The cat is thirsty and there is a loss of condition. One dose daily for 21 days.

**Conium 30C** - Use for injury to the eye especially in old cats. Hates bright light, eyes are watering, better in the dark. Dose daily for 4 days and see what happens.

**Cineraria Tincture** diluted 1 to 10. Can be highly beneficial for this condition. Use externally 2 to 3 drops twice daily for about 3 months. Most effective in traumatic cases.

**Senega 30C** - If the cat has a operation on the eye give this afterward at one dose a day for a week.

# Conjunctivitis

This is inflammation of the membrane on the inner eyelids and eyeball. This can be a acute or chronic condition. It can affect one or both eyes and is the major cause of reddened eyes. Even mild cases can get worse from the cat rubbing the irritated area. Can sometimes be associated with viral and bacterial infections along with allergies or a mechanical problem such as a blow or a foreign body such as a grass seed.

### Signs and Symptoms

At first the eyes may water and later the discharge thickens and may become brownish and mucoid. A deep red appearance to the eyes is present. There may be increased blinking, increased tear production, half closed eyes along with constant scratching around the eyes or rubbing of the face on hard objects or along the floor.

### Herbal Treatment

Eye Bright (Euphrasia) which is anti-inflammatory, astringent and anti-catarrhal is the main herb for use in eye problems used internally and externally. The whole plant is also nervine, tonic and very astringent. If a foreign object is in the eye use a piece of cotton wool soaked in warm water or lotion and wash around the eye and get a better look. For a little splinter in the eye or a hard to remove foreign body Castor Oil can be used for its drawing power as it has a good reputation for removing embedded objects and it will sooth the irritation at the same time. Put the oil in and leave overnight and the problem will usually be gone by the morning. Fennel is another good eye herb.

The eyes should be bathed with a 1 to 10 solution of Calendula and St John's Wort twice daily as this will with the Calendula give us a Antibacterial and Antifungal action and with St John's Wort we get a Antiviral and Antibacterial action. St John's Wort is good for pain. If you believe there is no underlying infection use Eye Bright or alternate back and forth. If you believe infection is the cause dose internally with Echinacea and Garlic.

## Homoeopathic Treatment

**Argent Nit 30C** - This remedy is useful for alleviating the condition. The animal is usually of a timid disposition showing signs of fear when approached. Dose daily for 7 days.

**Pulsatilla 6C -** Suitable for young animal of a affectionate disposition with changeable moods. Eye infection tend to become purulent due to secondary infection. Dose 3 times daily for 7 days.

**Ledum 6C -** If the condition is from the result of a scratch or stabbing injury to the eye. Dose 3 times daily for 7 days.

**Ruta Grav 1M -** Has a soothing effect on eye structures and will quickly help to ease the pain. Dose once daily for 7 days.

**Rhus Tox 1M -** Good for conjunctivitis in both eyes from allergy. There is intense irritation and the eyelids become swollen with maybe loss of hair around the margins. The animal is restless and appears to gain relief from moving place to place. Dose daily for 10 days.

**Hepar Sulph 1M** - Suited to the acute condition with a rapid purulent state. Extreme sensitivity to pain and touch. Dose twice daily for 6 days.

**Arnica 6C -** This is the remedy if the condition to the eye was caused by a blow leading to swelling and bruising. Dose 3 times daily for 5 days.

**Euphrasia 6C -** to 30C- Conjunctivitis after injury, eyes are hot, burning and watering, soreness, eye strain.  2 drops of tincture into a eye bath full of water gives relief to sore and wind burnt eyes. Use in potency as well.

**Symphytum 6C to 30C** - For blows to the eyeball itself, blunt injury trauma such as a tennis or squash ball.

**Merc Sol 30C** - For chronic states where the condition gets worse during the night. The discharge from the eye is greenish in colour. Dose 3 times weekly for 4 weeks.


# Glaucoma

In this condition the increasing internal fluid pressure of the eyeball can damage the retina and optic nerve and probably everything else. Lens dislocation can be a common cause for this condition.

## Signs and Symptoms

The constant swelling and bulging of the effected eye or eyes leading to eventual blindness. The cat will be in pain and shy away from light as this condition makes the pupils dilate.

## Herbal Treatment

This is a hard condition to treat with any of the Natural Remedies. Your main remedy is Bilberry which has a action of strengthening the capillaries in the eye. To this think of adding Rutin and Hesperidin which strengthen the walls of capillaries. Use Ginkgo Biloba to force the Bilberry into the head. Ginkgo is also a strong antioxidant so it will also add to the action we are trying to create. The idea is that if we can strengthen the capillaries and stop them from being leaky we can maybe reduce the pressure in the eye. If the condition has been brought on by trauma think of using Comfrey and Eyebright externally.

## Homoeopathic Treatment

**Aconitum 10M** - Give at the beginning of the problem to help give relief from the pain and stress. Repeat hourly for up to 3 doses.

**Apis 30C** - This may help the body to reabsorb some of the fluid in the eye. Dose twice daily for 14 days.

**Belladonna 1M** - As there will probably be throbbing and pulsation of the eye this remedy may help especially when the pupils are very dilated. Dose daily for 7 days.

**Spigelia 6C** - Pupils dilated, severe pain in and around eyes, eyes feel too large, photophobia, very sensitive to touch. Worse from touch, motion and noise.

**Phosphorus 200C -** In more long going cases this remedy should be considered. Dose 3 times weekly for 4 weeks.

## Chlamydial Infection
**See Infectious Diseases**

# Teeth

## Bad Breath
A healthy cat's breath doesn't smell.
Things to look for.
1. Is the cat drooling, if so it may have a mouth infection or gum disease.
2. Are the teeth stained? Tarter may be the cause leading to tooth decay.
3. Are the gums swollen or bleeding.
4. Gastric problems can cause bad breath, has it vomited?
5. Are there any mouth ulcers?, stomach ulcers?
6. Check for a broken tooth which may lead on to a abscess.
Regularly cleaning your cats teeth can be a good preventative and may save you a lot of money in the long run. Use a soft Childs tooth brush with a small head and warm slightly salted water. Start gradually and slowly, holding the mouth closed place the brush head in the mouths cheek and then the other side all the time talking softly to the cat. This is a long training process better started as a kitten. Never use human toothpaste.

## Gingivitis
This means inflammation of the gums.
### Signs and Symptoms
Bad breath is often the first symptom of diseases of the gums and teeth. The gums appear red and swollen especially close to the teeth and may be tender and painful. There may be excessive saliva and sometimes there may be ulceration. Yellow brown stains on the teeth where they meet the gums are a classic symptom. Sometimes the cat may lose its appetite as it is too painful to eat.

## Herbal Treatment

The best treatment is prevention as in brushing the teeth as mentioned above (good luck). Soft tinned food is the main culprit for this condition so give a more balanced diet. Internally think of Echinacea and Garlic not only to build the immunity but to deal with all the rubbish that the infection is putting in the blood stream. For external treatment think of Sage and Thyme either in tincture (dilute 1 to 10) or tea form (can be used for brushing teeth as well). If there is pain first use a tincture of St John's Wort diluted 1 to 5 for this is good for pains shooting along the nerve path ways which is commonly what teeth do especially damaged teeth. Save the Clove oil for last and severe pain (just try a tiny bit first and see what happens) as it is a terrible taste and smell and after prolonged use the smell will haunt you for life.

## Homoeopathic Treatment

**Merc Sol 6C -** Inflammation showing excessive saliva. There is a general dirty look to the mouth. Symptoms worse during the night. Dose 3 times daily for 10 days.

**Merc Iod Rub 30C -** More for inflammation on the left side of the mouth. Dose 3 times daily for 7 days.

**Merc Iod Flav 30C -** More for inflammation on the right side of the mouth. Dose 3 times daily for 7 days.

**Borax 6C -** Ulceration is present when this remedy is indicated. Salivation is excessive. Dose twice daily for 14 days.

**Mecr Corr 30C -** For this mercury the symptoms are much more severe than the others. Dose twice daily for 7 days.

# Infectious Diseases

## Feline Viral Rhinotracheitis (Herpes virus)

Symptoms are sneezing, coughing, eyes and nose discharge, fever, drooling, lack of appetite, termination of pregnancy (abortion). Has a 2 to 10 day incubation period after this it produces inflammation of the eyes, nose, windpipe along with the resultant discharges. The Cat becomes apathetic and feverish, loses its appetite and sneezes continually. Discharges from eyes and nose become thicker and purulent and sometimes the cat develops painful ulcers on its tongue. This is usually a severe infection of longer then a week's duration and can be fatal especially to kittens and the elderly cat. Recovered animals can become carriers. The temperature can rise to 105 F in severe cases.

## Herbal Treatment

With infectious diseases as fast acting and as serious as this use high doses of Vitamin C immediately, you could crush up the pills or use the powdered form that you can buy at health shops, use at least 1000mg a day. Those of you who have Troy's injectable Vitamin C can give 5cc morning and night.

It would be best to fast the cat that is if the cat is not doing so already especially at the beginning stages and it is not wise to give food while they have a fever so try to wait till the fever breaks, meanwhile you could give the cat honey and water so they remain hydrated and have some nutrition, use this to get your herbal formula into them. Use the immune boosting and infection fighting herbs like Echinacea, Garlic and Myrrh constantly throughout the illness and add to them other herbs as the symptoms change. Yarrow would be herb to add to the immune boosters for the fever and would also help with the discharges as its other actions are antiseptic and astringent. Other astringents that may be useful here are Golden Rod and Eyebright (Euphrasia) Try when you select your herbs to get them to overlap and cover other symptoms in their actions as I have done with Yarrow.

## Homoeopathic Treatment

**Aconitum 30C** - Give as early as possible where it can sometimes stop the problem from developing further.

**Pulsatilla 30C** - This remedy has been described as the nearest one can get to a constitutional remedy for a cat, while many cats do indeed respond well to it there are other remedies that can fit the symptoms. Usually a affectionate animal showing variable symptoms and alteration of moods, discharges are copious and bland. It is worth considering in the early stages of this infection, dose 3 times daily for 5 days.

**Ant Tart 30C** - Useful if broncho- pneumonic symptoms develop, coughing is of the moist type and expectoration is muco-purulent though scanty, prefers to lay on the right side, dose once daily for 10 days.

**Phosphorus 200C** - This deep acting remedy may be needed when involvement of the nasal septum and turbinate bones develops. Caries or necrosis of these structures calls for this remedy associated with violent sneezing of blood stained muco purulent mucous. It may also be indicated in bronchial conditions when the patient coughs up blood stained mucous. Haemorrhage is a keynote of this remedy along with its destructive effect on various body systems. One dose 3 times weekly.

**Kali Bich 200C** - When this remedy is indicated the nasal and bronchial secretions are thick, tough and yellowish. Expectoration and sneezing show little mucous, the remedy is indicated when ulceration of the nasal septum develops. One dose twice weekly for 6 weeks.

**Silicea 200C** - If treatment is delayed and secondary involvement of the eye structures develop eg keratitis this remedy may help. It will speed the resolution of early scar tissue and remove the cloudiness and opacity which is apparent at this phase of the disease. One dose 3 times weekly for 6 weeks.

# Feline Calici Virus

This viral disease shows a variety of symptoms depending on the severity of the infection and the structures of the body or the systems that are involved.

## Sign and Symptoms

The incubation period is about 5 to 7 days, temperature rise, followed by lethargy, poor appetite, watery discharge from the eyes and nose and dribbling from the mouth, ulcers on the tongue. Salivation is profuse with large strings of saliva being seen, the temperature can rise to 105 F. The nasal septum becomes ulcerated leading to bouts of muco purulent sneezing. Pneumonia is a common complication. Recovery normally takes place in a week. Infection can be from very mild to fatal. Good nursing is very important, clean away discharge from eyes and nose. Inhalations may help with breathing.

## Herbal Treatment

Is very similar to Feline Viral Rhinotracheitis. Look in the respiratory section and match symptoms to the herbs used there.

## Homoeopathic Treatment

**Aconitum 30C** - Give as early as possible where it can sometimes stop the problem from developing further.

**Merc Sol 3oC-** Indicated when salivation is excessive, has a good action on the mouth, there is a general dirty look to the mouth and the patient is worse from sun rise to sunset, Give 1 dose daily for 14 days.

**Kali Bich 200C** - When this remedy is indicated the nasal and bronchial secretions are thick, tough and yellowish. Expectoration and sneezing show little mucous, the remedy is indicated when ulceration of the nasal septum develops. One dose twice weekly for 6 weeks.

**Phosphorus 200C** - This deep acting remedy may be needed when involvement of the nasal septum and turbinate bones develops. Caries or necrosis of these structures calls for this remedy associated with violent sneezing of blood stained muco purulent mucous. It may also be indicated in bronchial conditions when the patient coughs up blood stained mucous. Haemorrhage is a keynote of this remedy along with its destructive effect on various body systems. Should also prove helpful if Pneumonia sets in, there is usually rapid involvement of lung tissue with severe difficulty in breathing, expectoration is scanty and blood stained. One dose 3 times weekly.

# Feline Infectious Peritonitis

FIP is caused by a virus infecting the stomach area but also affecting the adjacent organs. The condition is actually made worse by the cats own immune system which speeds up the progress of the disease. FIP occurs in two forms wet and dry. Cats of 6 months to 2 years old are most susceptible though older cats can be infected to. It is also more common in pure bred cats and in cats living in a multi cat environment. The cause is a virus and after a incubation period of up to 14 days or longer the cats initial temperature rise can be up to 106 F. Other signs are lethargy, poor appetite, weight loss, swollen abdomen, fever, if the peritoneum is effected it produces fluid which causes the abdomen to swell while if the pleura is effected the produced liquid pushes on the lungs causing laboured breathing. There can be involvement of one or both of the eyes, with the most notable change being in eye colour. If the brain is effected a variety of symptoms appear.  Cats with this disease usually die within 6 weeks.

## Herbal Treatment

Echinacea, Garlic and Myrrh because of their immune building and their anti-viral actions. Add other herbs as and when are needed to cover the other symptoms. Go into the different sections to find the symptoms in the different systems.

**Vitamin C** - Use sodium ascorbate acid powder to bowel tolerance, start with one eighth of a teaspoon 3 to 4 times daily and gradually increase dosage amount in food till the poops are runny then back off the dosage a bit. If the pet is not eating well then dilute the powder in half a teaspoon of water and syringe inside the pets mouth 3 to 4 times daily.

## Homoeopathic Treatment

**Cantharis 6C** - Can be of use for peritoneal cases especially the painful inflammations.

**Apis 6c** - Apis is used for various types of swelling and inflammation. Apis is a quick acting remedy for inflammations especially those ones with oedema and lots of swelling which is its main use. Symptoms are swelling with oedema which makes the effected parts look shiny, red and puffy, the swollen parts feel soggy and waterlogged, a fever that develops rapidly but without thirst, extreme restlessness and fidgeting, an irritable nature and perhaps jealous, cool air and cold compresses relieve the symptoms. Pains are burning and stinging, animals seek cold surface to lie on, swollen eyelids, may be swollen ears, may be blood in the urine, Symptoms get worse from heat and improve in the open air and from cold bathing.. If this remedy is a close match use it in high potency.

**Aconitum 30C** - Give as early as possible where it can sometimes stop the problem from developing further.

**Lycopodium 12C** - A prominent liver remedy, inability to eat much at any one time, very little food appears to satisfy, all symptoms aggravated in the late afternoon and early evening, a good remedy for the old and for lean animals, premature greying of the coat could be another sign for this remedy, stools are generally hard. For the more chronic cases showing indigestion and flatulence, oedema of the abdomen.

## Feline Urological Syndrome (FUS)

This is a inflammation of the bladder and the urethra together with the formation of crystals and stones. In females the urethra is shorter and wider so obstruction with stones or sand is rare while in males the urethra is long, has a bend  and is narrower so for males obstruction of the urethra is a lot more common. This condition can be fatal in male cats.

**Causes** - Infection, alkaline urine, excessive magnesium in the diet, restricted access to water, excessive dry food, restricted access to the place where the cat usually urinates causing the cat to retain urine for long periods.

**Symptoms** - Squatting frequently, straining to urinate, licking around penis or vulva, urinating in unusual places, crying in pain especially when picked up, lethargic, swollen abdomen, shock, not eating, end of penis if protruding may be red to bluish in colour.

**Treatment** - If there is a blockage this can be fatal, take to the vet.

Prevention can be achieved by acidifying the urine because inflammation and crystal forming occur more frequently in alkaline urine. As magnesium is found in the most common crystals another approach can be to reduce the dietary intake of magnesium which can be done by feeding it no more than 20% of dry food in the diet or take it off dry food completely for a while. Increased fluid intake flushes out the system and can be achieved by adding water to food or a bit of salt to make the cat thirsty.

**Herbal Treatment -** Cranberry juice if the cat will drink it ,see the conditions in the appropriate section.

**Homoeopathic Treatment** - Causticum, Cantharis, see the conditions in the appropriate section.

# Feline Chlamydial Infection

The cause is infection with the bacteria Chlamydial Psittaci. The disease is spread from the discharges of other infected cats. This now seems to be spreading faster than before. Most common in young, 1 to 9 months of age. Diagnosis is from blood or discharge test and if the results are positive antibiotics will be used for treatment. If the infection is not treated quickly it can lead on to digestive and genital problems affecting queens in later life.

## Signs and Symptoms

The eyes and upper respiratory system are affected leading to rhinitis of a acrid nature and sneezing. Eye symptoms are prominent with conjunctivitis usually being severe with a gummy sticky discharge which sometimes leads to the eyelids sticking together. The temperature can remain normal. Usually severe in kittens.

## Herbal Treatment

Herbs to consider are Echinacea and Garlic for the main antibacterial attack and Elder, Golden Rod and Agrimony for the flu like symptoms. Consider Eyebright (works well with Golden Rod and Fennel) added to a internal formula and you can also use it as a lotion maybe mixed with Calendula for wiping and cleaning the external discharge away.

## Homoeopathic Treatment

**Argentum Nit 30C -** A good remedy for conjunctival problems, purulent involvement is common. Chronic cases may show corneal ulceration with which this remedy will help. The cat may show fear of being handled by trembling and trying to escape. Dose daily for 10 days.

**Graphites 6C** - The leading symptoms art stickiness of discharges especially in regards to the eye. Eye lids are red and swollen, may feel better in the dark. For severe cases with closure of the eye. Dose 3 times daily for 7 days.

**Kali Bich 200C** - Nasal discharges are thick and yellow and difficult to expel. Dose twice weekly for 4 weeks.

**Phosphorus 200C** - Consider if the deeper structures of the eye become involved. This remedy has a profound action on the eyes and also on the nasal structures. Here the nasal discharge may be streaked with blood. Dose twice weekly for 6 weeks.

**Chlamydia Nosode 30C** - This disease Nosode can be used with the other remedies. Dose daily for 10 days.

# Herbal Supplement
## Introduction to Herbal Medicine

Herbal Medicine has been in use and developed continuously since the beginning of time. It mainly evolved from observations from what plants did and the affects they had on people along with their animals. There is also what they call the Doctrine of Signatures which works like this, that flower really looks like a eye, maybe it helps sore eyes? I'll give it a try as my eyes are so sore and red. You know my eye really feels a lot better now, I think I will call that plant Eye Bright (Euphrasia) and tell my friends all about it especially my Dad who gets sore eyes to. In this way hundreds of plants were identified that have a medical action and no doubt there were also a lot of casualties. The next great leap in herbal medicine was the Roman Empire of 2000 years ago. The Great Armies of Rome all had their own Medical Corps with Doctors, Battle Surgeons and Orderlies. It was these men who already had the knowledge of the Greeks that started to put together the best medical manuals in the world while at the same time started developing and using medical instruments and tools some of which are still used today. As the Romans conquered the known world more medicines and knowledge were found and assimilated. The next great leap was modern Chemistry which allowed us to see exactly what herbs were made up of and what parts of the herb causes its medical action. Drug companies have made billions of Dollars from this information as they find the main active ingredient and then make a synthetic version of it, one good example that we all know of is Valium which is the synthetic version of the active ingredient from the herb Valerian. Leaving aside the Drug Companies let's see how Chemistry changed the way that modern herbalists think. Modern science allows us to now know what Actions our herbs perform on the body so we shall carry on using Valerian as a example and see what Medical Actions Valerian has on the body.

The Actions of Valerian are Sedative, Hypnotic (sleep inducing), Anti Spasmodic (stops twitches, cramps etc), Hypotensive (lowers Blood Pressure) and Carminative (calms and relaxes the tummy). Herbalists call Valerian the Herbal Tranquillizer and if you look at the above you can see why for if you can't sleep and your blood pressures up along with a gurgling tummy and an eye constantly twitching you definitely need to be calmed down.

The modern herbalist is trained to think in actions. There are many reasons for this but the main ones are to stop them from just using a handful of their favourite herbs and to train the mind to work in the method of thinking in actions that are needed. If we start thinking in the actions that are needed for a patient it makes us consider the problem in far more depth than just using our favourite herb and it forces our thinking to be far more holistic by taking in consideration the whole of the patient not just the part or the system we wish to treat. Let's take a look at thinking in actions. The animal has a cough, but when it coughs it can't stop and the cough sounds a bit like whooping cough. The animal also sounds a little hoarse and the temperature is also elevated. The actions that come into mind for this are expectorant for the cough, antispasmodics for the whooping quality of the cough and demulcents to sooth the sore throat. These are the obvious actions and we can add many more if we wish such as immune boosters for acute diseases, diaphoretics to reduce the temperature and prevent a fever and the list goes on. Next we look at how Herbal Actions are used in making Herbal Formulas.

Another point to make before we go to the formula making is that Professional Herbalists use Herbs in the form of Tinctures (water and alcohol solutions) as this allows them to mix formulas in any proportions that they like and also allows long term storage without spoiling.

# Making Herbal Formulas

You should never have more the 5 Herbs in a herbal formula otherwise you start to loose track of what you are doing and how the formula is changing the symptoms. Always try to keep things simple. One of the herbs in the formula is used to force the formula into the body, to keep it simple we will only use three; they are Licorice, Ginger and Cayenne.

As an example let's use a animal with a cough.  After further study of the case we decide that this is a Acute Disease for it came on quick and is fast acting not slow like a Chronic Disease. Listening to the animals cough we decide that it is a dry cough and upon looking at the animals nose we can't see any mucus. Let's list the actions to consider.

**Expectorants -** Licorice, Aniseed, Fennel, Garlic and Mullein
**Antispasmodics** - Aniseed and Fennel
**Demulcents** - Licorice and Coltsfoot
**Immune Boosters** - Echinacea
**Anti Bacterial and Virals** - Garlic and Echinacea

Out of the above I would choose Licorice, Echinacea, Garlic, Aniseed and Fennel. I would make the formula in this strength.

### Formula
**Licorice - 20%**
**Garlic - 15%**
**Echinacea - 15%**
**Aniseed - 30%**
**Fennel - 20%**

Look these herbs up in the herbal and consider why I used them, there are three obvious ones for Licorice alone with the first being to force the assimilation of the formula into the body, second is its expectorant action and third is its demulcent action in case the throat is sore and raw. Next time you see a little kid eating heaps of licorice get them to open their mouth and look at their tongue which will be going black from the Licorice along with the throat etc and know that you are looking at the demulcent action of Licorice working by coating and soothing.

The most important reason that you use the Actions Method for Herbal Prescribing is so that you can concentrate the Actions which are most needed for example, if it's a Bacterial infection concentrate on the Anti Bacterials, if it's a Viral infection concentrate on the Anti Virals, hopefully you are now beginning to see the importance of working in actions for if you don't concentrate a large part of the battle on the causes you may have lost the battle from the start.

Read through all the Actions listed in Herbal Actions at the end of each body system in the book and then do a study in depth of at least five Actions of your choice making the first two the Anti Bacterials and Anti Virals. Start trying to train your mind into thinking in Actions.

## How to Make Herbal Tinctures

Tinctures are made by steeping the Herb plant material in a mixture of alcohol and water. Alcohol is usually always used at a strength of 45%. The alcohol in this mixture will extract all the essential oils from the herb while the water will extract all that is water soluble, so between the both we are getting most of the medicinal properties out of the herb. The proportions of herb to liquid are usually 1 part herb to 5 parts liquid. So find a suitable container (I use a big one litre preserving jar with a good sealing lid) and put into it 100grams of your chosen herb and to that add 500mls of our 45% solution of alcohol. Seal the lid and shake well for about a minute. Leave the jar on the window sill so the sun can shine on the jar for two weeks. The jar must be shaken for at least a minute every day.

After 2 weeks open and filter the contents of the jar. I use a large pouring jug into which I place a funnel and then place a coffee filter in the funnel and pour the jar contents through the funnel being careful not to let too much herb spill into the filter and block it up. When you get to the bottom of the jar you can crush the herb in your fist so as to extract the last of the liquid.

After this is completed you then get your chosen storage bottle, put a funnel into its neck followed by a coffee filter and then filter the jug into the bottle. Remember the solution should always be double filtered

Next we label the bottle, put the date, name and proportions eg 1 to 5 also state the recommended dose. Store in a cool and dark place. Most Professional Homoeopaths and Herbalists have access to pure alcohol so for them it is fairly easy to make tinctures while for the lay person they will probably have a hard time. A alternative is to use Vodka as strong as you can find it or find a way to twist the authorities arm into giving alcohol at 45%. Don't even try to get pure alcohol as it is dangerous and can turn people blind and they won't give it to you.

## How to Make Infusions

Infusions are a bit like making a cup of tea except we don't use milk. Infusions are used for the soft parts of the herb such as the flowers, leaves and fine twigs. The proportions for infusions are 1 to 20 eg 1 part herb to 20 parts water. Infusions are used for the more water soluble herbs. Infusions can be made from a single herb or from a combination of herbs and may be drunk hot or cold. The water should be just off the boil before being poured on the herb and if you are making a infusion of a herb strong in essential oils such as Peppermint always cover the top of the cup  to stop the essential oils from escaping in steam while the infusion is brewing. Allow up to 10 minutes to brew. It is best to make herbal teas fresh each day. You can experiment on yourself by getting Chamomile and Peppermint tea bags from the supermarket. Use honey as a sweetener.

# How to Make Decoctions

Decoctions are used for the more hard woody substances of the herb such as barks, berries or roots. The process of decoction is far more vigorous then  infusion as it involves heating the plant material in cold water, bringing it to the boil and simmering for 20 to 40 minutes. The finished ratio for decoctions is again 1 part herb to 20 parts water, remember to add more water at the beginning so you wind up with the 1 to 20 after steam loss. This form of preparation is no good for the herbs that are high in essential oils as these will all be lost in the steam.

# How to Make Poultices

Poultices are used to sooth, irritate or draw impurities from the skin so choose your required plants by the actions you need. A Poultice is used to apply a remedy to the skin with moist heat and slight pressure. To prepare a poultice bruise or crush the fresh medicinal parts of the herb you are using into a pulpy mass and add a little hot water if needed. If using dried herb moisten the material by mixing with a hot soft adhesive substance such as moist flower and cornmeal or as they did in the past a mixture of bread and milk. This can be done to the fresh herb if you want as well. For ease of application to the skin it is best to spread the mixture on cheese cloth and fold to the appropriate size or shape required. The cloth also helps by retaining the moisture and even allows you to tie it gently the  affected area. Moisten the cloth with hot water periodically when and if needed. Hot water bottles can also be used to keep the poultice warm. Always keep some cloth between the skin when using irritant plants such as mustard and always wash the skin thoroughly after use.

# Dosage for Forms of Herbal Medicines

Herbs can be given to animals in several different forms depending on what best suites the herb, the ailment, and the condition of the animal and of what is available at the time and then most importantly the expense. I prefer using liquid to medicate in tinctures, extracts or infusion form even though there can be some controversy over the alcohol. The reason for this is that liquid spreads through the intestines a greater distance then the dry form which insures maximum absorption and uptake. Juliette de Bairacli Levy uses mainly infusions made from one handful of the fresh herb or 2 heaped tablespoons of the dried herb to one pint of cold water slowly heated and simmered for a while not boiled. She uses infusions because cellulose is not easily digested in carnivore animals though she does use some herbal powders.

**Herbal Tincture Dose** - Cats are sensitive to alcohol so only give them about 3 drops of tincture at a time in water and maybe mixed with honey so as to disguise the taste, a syringe plunger is a easy way to dose them. This is a fairly low and safe dose and can be repeated about three times a day.  Always go by what the maker of the tincture says because all herbs are not the same strength some are very strong with a good example being Poke Root. For animal with a bad liver or who just can't take alcohol you can do what we do to human Alcoholic, mix the tincture with very hot water and the water will evaporate the alcohol away. These days you can now buy glycetracts which use glycerin instead of alcohol for extraction.

**Infusion Dose** - One teaspoon up to three times a day is a fairly safe dose but always take into consideration the strength of the herb.

**Herbal Extract** - Are alcohol based and about the strongest herbal preparation you can get as they nearly extract everything from the herb. Generally the strength is every ml should be equivalent to one gram of the herb. Used and dosed the same as tinctures but the dose will always be less then what is used in a tincture. From this try to work out if the extra price is worth it. Supplier should give dosage.

**Tincture** - Is a weaker then Herbal Extracts but also made from alcohol. Dilute the appropriate number of drops in water for treatment. Supplier should give dosage.

**Infusion** - A infusion is like making a cup of tea out of the flowers and leaves and other soft parts of the herb. Add boiling water and cover so as all the essential oils don't escape in the steam and leave for 20 minutes.

**Decoction** - Usually made from the root, bark or seed and is simmered for a while to extract the medicinal properties. Usually dosed the same as infusions.

**Powdered** - These are usually made from roots and bark and given in doses from a teaspoon to tablespoon. These can also be infused and turned into a tea.

**Note** - Always be guided by the recommended dose of the individual herb instead of working in generals.

## Calculating Correct Herbal Doses for Animals

**Cats** - 1/8 to 1/6 the dose for an adult human.

**Dogs** - Correspond to adult human dose according to weight.

**Horse** - 8 to 16 times the dose for an adult human.

**Goats** - 2 times the dose for an adult human.

**Sheep** - 1 1/2 times the dose for an adult human.

**Cow -** 12 to 24 times the dose for an adult human.

**Swine -** 1 to 3 times the dose for an adult human.

Not all herbs are of the same strength so for this reason it is a good idea to always look at the human dose and if this dose seems to be lower than normal, if it is do your research into why. It might be a good idea to have a look at the herb Poke Root just to see what a strong herb looks like and can do.

**Warning** - For cats beware of the aspirin like herbs like Meadowsweet and Willow Bark, only use Garlic in small doses mixed with other herbs. Generally herbs in a well thought out formula tend to buffer each other and minimise the side effects.

## Good Cat Herbs

These are herbs that are fairly safe for use and have a history of cat use and most importantly they should be easy for you to find. There are lots more herbs that you can use but get used to these ones first and slowly expand.

## Agrimony

**Actions** - Astringent, cholagogue, diuretic, vulnerary, tonic

Used as a remedy for jaundice, it should be given to fasting animal as a drench or finely cut and mixed with bran, it is also a valuable astringent to stem bleeding and is a remedy for sore throats. Sprains are aided by a lotion made by boiling one handful of chopped Agrimony in one quart of brew made from wheaten bran. The combination of astringency and of bitter tonic properties make this a powerful herb for the digestive system. This is a good and gentle remedy for the young.

**Uses -** Diarrhoea in the young, mucous colitis, spring tonic, indigestion, urinary incontinence and cystitis, as a gargle for sore throats and laryngitis and as a ointment or lotion for wounds and bruises.

**For Cats and Dogs -** Sore throats, Tonsillitis, infections of the mouth, Ailments of the lungs, stomach, liver kidney and bladder particularly cirrhosis of the liver and  jaundice, it helps rheumatism, poor digestion and back pain and is excellent for enlargement of the heart and disorders of the spleen. Infusions, decoctions, ointments.

**Cautions** - Not to be used during Pregnancy

# Alfalfa

Known also as Lucerne.  Rich in nitrates and vitamins is a good tonic food and a kidney cleanser. Excellent for all animals and poultry. It is a healthy and nutritious source of chlorophyll, beta carotene, calcium, and the vitamins D, E and K. Fodder, tonic, nervine, aids in healing allergies, arthritis, morning sickness, peptic ulcers, stomach ailments and bad breath, removes poisons from the body, neutralizes acids, is a excellent blood purifier and thinner, improves appetite and aids in the assimilation of protein, calcium and other nutrients.

**Cat** - Half a teaspoon of alfalfa sprouts mixed into meals. Stops them from wanting to eat grass.

# Calendula

**Actions -** Anti-inflammatory, astringent, vulnerary, anti-fungal, cholagogue, emmenagogue.
A good cancer herb which also brings great relief to inflammation of the liver. It purifies the blood so stimulating the circulation and bringing swift healing to wounds. One of the best Vulnerary herbs for external use.

**Uses** - Cuts, grazes, infected sores, fungal infections, any skin inflammations, regulates the oil production of the skin so is good for acne, to stop bleeding, bruises and sprains, skin ulcers and minor burns and scolds, healing, soothing, anti-microbial. Use as a lotion to clean wounds, one of our main germacides for wounds and if Hypericum is added to the lotion you may prevent tetanus as well.

**Caution** - Calendula closes wounds rapidly so make sure they are very clean and no foreign bodies remain.

## Chamomile

**Actions** - Stomachic, antispasmodic, anti-allergy, sedative, anti-inflammatory, carminative, analgesic and anti-septic.

It is a famed blood cleanser and pain reducer, reduces tumours (poultice), remedy for female ailments, inflamed gums, use for blood and skin disorders, aches and pains, external and internal inflammations, delayed menstruation, acid uterus and all female ailments, cleanser and toner of the digestive tract, expels worms and parasites, improves and helps appetite. This herb is also anti-allergy.

**Uses** - Indigestion, colic, diarrhoea, teething children, anxiety, insomnia, **nervous upsets,** slowing down hyperactive children, flatulence. Good all round tonic for the nervous system especially for nervous animals.

**Cats and Dogs** - Good for kittens and puppies, administer in all cases of stomach pain, wind, upsets, gastritis, restlessness and fever. Can be given also for all abdominal and uterine disorders, inflammation of the testicles, wounds, toothaches, eruptions and as a steam bath for colds and feline respiratory diseases. Fevers, back and rheumatic pains are eased by the tea and regular massages with the oil. The infusion is good for nervous disorders and a tonic for kidney and urinary tract problems

## Cat Nip - Cat Mint - Carminative, antispasmodic, diaphoretic, sedative, astringent.

Cats eat the plant and give themselves a massage in it in order to benefit from its medicinal properties. It will sometimes cause cats to grow pensive and dreamy. It is a digestive plant that will heal colic, flatulence and internal inflammation. It stops coughs and is a gentle efficient pain killer.

## Cleavers

**Actions** - Alterative, diuretic, anti-inflammatory, tonic, astringent, lymphatic tonic.

A lymphatic tonic with alterative and diuretic actions which can be used in a wide range of problems where the lymphatic system is involved. The plant is very rich in minerals and silica, gives good strong texture to the hair of animals and the shells of eggs. All animals eat it and poultry especially seek it hence its popular name of goose grass. Good for skin ailments.

**Uses** - Tonic, eczema, abscesses and tumours, cancerous growths, swollen glands, tonsillitis, psoriasis, cystitis.

**Cats and Dogs** - Cleavers is a great purifier of the kidneys, pancreas and spleen. Disorders of the uterus, the lymphatic system and the skin are helped by this herb. The fresh juice applied to cases of feline acne and eczema quickly alleviates the problem as do regular washings of the infected areas with cleavers tea. Washes can also be used on wounds and abscesses. Internal treatment can be used for epilepsy, anaemia, dropsy, nervous complaints and constriction of the vocal cords. Toms suffering from a blocked bladder will be greatly helped by a regular dose of cleavers as the tea dissolves gravely deposits in the bladder. Cancer of the tongue and mouth and other cancerous growths are helped.

## Coltsfoot

**Actions** - Expectorant, anti-spasmodic, demulcent, anti-catarrhal, diuretic.

The Latin name means banish cough.. Coltsfoot combines a soothing expectorant action with a anti spasmodic action. There are useful zinc levels in this plant. Consider this herb in any respiratory problem.

**Uses** - Coughs, pneumonia, asthma, pleurisy, TB, sedative powers in epilepsy, chronic or acute bronchitis, emphysema, cystitis.

**Externally** - A poultice is used for abscess, ulcers, boils, earache and toothache.

**Cats and Dogs** - Most particularly a chest herb with powerful expectorant and anti-inflammatory properties. Excellent for cases of bronchitis, bronchial asthma, pleurisy, Feline Respiratory Disease and chest problems that accompany a range of feline fungal diseases. It can be given with honey and lemon when coughing is a persistent problem. Can be used as a poultice for non-healing wounds. Ear infections can be helped by the fresh juice.

## Comfrey

**Actions** - Demulcent, Astringent, Expectorant, Vulnerary.

Once widely cultivated as a fodder plant, sheep and cows eat it greedily, the impressive wound healing powers of comfrey are partially due to allantoin which stimulates cell proliferation and speeds the healing process inside and out.

**Uses** - Its old name is knit bone and that describes well what it does. Comfrey also guards against scar tissue from developing incorrectly, all internal haemorrhages including uterine, reunion of wound and fractures, internal ulcers, ruptures, pulmonary problems, bronchitis, irritable cough, ulcerative colitis, skin ulcers and varicose veins.

**Cats and Dogs -** One of the best wound and bone setting herbs. The tincture is effective of curing rheumatism and swollen joints even where arthritis has caused extensive damage. The tincture has been used for paralysis. Massage well into the joints and muscles of the affected parts. Where paralysis is due to shock, dislocation or sprain apply as a poultice. A cold infused tisane prepared overnight from the roots is good for digestive ailments, bronchitis, internal bleeding in the stomach, lungs or bowels, pleurisy and internal ulcers.

## Corn Silk

**Actions** - Diuretic, demulcent, tonic, cystitis, prostrate.

A soothing diuretic that is helpful in any irritation of the membranes of the urinary system. Combined with other herbs in the treatment of cystitis, urethritis and prostatitis. Cleanses and soothes the urinary system.

**Cats and Dogs** - Good for the treatment of obesity and as it is a powerful diuretic it can be used for all complaints of the bladder and kidneys especially stones, edema, fluid in the heart, nephritis, cystitis, renal colic, and rheumatism.

## Dandelion

**Actions** - Diuretic, cholagogue, anti-rheumatic, laxative, tonic.

The herb is blood cleansing and tonic, it has a important effect on the hepatic system and is a supreme jaundice curative herb, the leaves strengthen the enamel of the teeth and the white   juices of the freshly crushed stem dissolves warts, the plant is well grazed by goats, horses will take quantities of the leaves when cut and well mixed with bran, excellent for anaemia because it is high in iron, calcium, copper and vitamins, useful in kidney and bladder problems, skin eruptions, sluggish blood flow, weak arteries, all liver complaints, jaundice, constipation, gallbladder problems and rheumatism.

**Cats and Dogs** - A good liver herb especially for gall bladder complaints. It can be used for eczema and feline miliary dermatitis and is a healing tonic for the spleen. Internal digestive toning and cleansing along with metabolic disorders.

## Elder

**Actions** - Expectorant, diaphoretic, flu, hay fever, sinusitis, purgative, flowers are anti-catarrhal.

Most animals will graze on elder. Used for the treatment of all gastric, hepatic, and pulmonary ailment, all fevers, skin disorders especially scabies and ring worm, externally as a insecticide. Elder is mainly used to treat colds, flu, dry coughs, sinusitis and catarrh.

## Feverfew

**Actions** - Anti-inflammatory, vasodilator, relaxant, digestive bitter, uterine stimulant.

It is one of the most important aids for female ailments the plant exerting remarkable powers over the uterus, the whole plant is used. Has a good reputation for headaches, may help with arthritis when it is in the inflammatory stage. Digestive aid and tonic, inflamed or weak uterus and uterine and vaginal ulcers, abortion, difficult labour, retained afterbirth, arthritis, inflammations.

## Fenugreek

**Actions** - Expectorant, demulcent tonic, galactagogue, lymphatic drainage.

The plant possesses highly aromatic seeds having a powerful disinfectant and emollient lubricant properties. The feeding value of these is about equal to linseed. It is one of the great fattening herbs. The perfect sister herb for garlic enhancing all its powers. Very tonic and eagerly sought by all animals. Rich in vitamins and nitrates, calcium and phosphorus. The whole plant is used. Good for all gastric weaknesses and ailments, nerves and neuralgia, female ailments including failing milk supply, allergies, bronchitis, anaemia, bruises, colitis, coughs, diabetes, fever, flu, hay fever, headache, migraines, lung problems, sinus congestion, ulcers, reduces inflammation.

## Ginger

**Actions** - Carminative, diaphoretic, circulatory stimulant, anti-inflammatory.

Ginger is warming and disinfectant and contains many healing virtues. Has a good action on the circulatory system and inflammations of the joints. Can be added to a formula to force assimilation and good for travel sickness.

## Garlic

**Actions** - Anti septic, antiviral, diaphoretic, cholagogue, anti-spasmodic, hypotensive.

The plant is rich in volatile oil and sulphur and because of its remarkable penetrating, disinfecting and mucous expelling powers garlic is a valuable basic remedy for the treatment of all ailments in which the cleansing of the blood stream and expulsion of mucous accumulations is required. Garlic is extremely effective in dissolving and cleansing cholesterol from the blood stream, it stimulates the digestive tract, kills worms, parasites and harmful bacteria, normalizes blood pressure, reduces fever, gas and cramps. Use for all infections, coughs, colds, flu, bronchitis, all fevers, pulmonary conditions, gastric and skin complaints, rheumatism, all worms and also liver fluke, mange, ringworm, ticks and lice.

**Caution** - There is a lot of contradictory information out there about garlic for dogs saying it causes anaemia. Sort term use would be alright.

## Golden Rod

**Actions** - Anti-inflammatory, antiseptic, diaphoretic, flu, anti-catarrhal, cystitis, diaphoretic, carminative, diuretic, astringent, tonic, hypotensive.

It is famed as a wound herb, is a important remedy for female disorders, all cattle eat it and it brings them into good appetite and gives bloom, the whole plant is used, traditionally used for inflammation, upper respiratory catarrh, use with other herbs for influenza, flatulent dyspepsia, as a urinary anti-inflammatory and anti-septic, cystitis, urethritis and also used for urinary stones. This herb is also used for arthritis.

**Uses** - A powerful digestive aid, treatment of jaundice, kidney problems.

**Externally** - For wounds, to stop bleeding, cleansing gangrenous conditions.

**Cat and Dog** - The blossoms are gathered to treat intestinal ulceration and bleeding of the intestines as well as dysentery, vomiting and flatulence. Leaves and flowers are used for kidney complaints as well as urinary and bladder problems.

**Dosage of infusion** - Give a cat 1/2 teaspoon orally or in food 2 x daily.

# Horehound

**Actions** - Expectorant, antispasmodic, bitter.

Is one of the most important pectoral herbs a famed cough and throat remedy, the bitter action stimulates the flow of bile and thus improves digestion. Use for the treatment of cough, pneumonia, pleurisy, bronchitis, atrophy of the lungs, ear disorders, diarrhoea, inflammation of the liver, jaundice.

# Horsetail

**Actions** - Astringent, diuretic, enlarged prostrate, incontinence.

Goats eat the plant but it is not a good food for cows, excellent astringent for the genito-urinary system reducing bleeding and healing wounds thanks to its high silica content, inflammation of the prostrate, tones and astringes the urinary system making it a good remedy for incontinence and bed wetting. Use for kidney stones as the high silica content erodes stones. May speed up the healing of bone, flesh and cartilage due to its high mineral content.

**Uses -** Nasal haemorrhage, laryngitis, intestinal ulcer, inflammation of the uterus, vagina and bladder, dysentery, enlarged anal glands, obesity, dropsy, a strong dose dissolves stones in the bladder.

**Caution** - If used over a long period it may decrease vitamin B1.

**Cats and Dogs** - Good for stopping internal bleeding and vomiting of blood. Used for kidney and bladder problems, gravel and stones.

# Hyssop

**Actions** - Expectorant, antispasmodic, sedative, carminative, diaphoretic.

A important plant in pectoral complaints because it removes mucous accumulations and also tones up the membranes and fortifies the whole system. Is a mild vermifuge the Nordic countries use it as a vermifuge for delicate lambs and kids. Coughs, bronchitis, chronic catarrh, colds and flu's, anxiety states, hysteria, petit mal. Use for the treatment of cough, sore throat, pneumonia, pleurisy, worms, eye disorders, conjunctivitis.

# Ladys Mantle

**Actions -** Astringent, emmenagogue, anti-inflammatory, diuretic.

This herb has a affinity to the womb where it helps with pain, bleeding and getting the cycle back to normal. Horses, goats and sheep seek out the herb, the plant is tonic and an important fortifier for the blood and walls of the arteries, it is a old herbal remedy for diabetes, reduces period pains and excessive bleeding, diarrhoea, sores, ulcers a good menopause herb.

**Uses -** Treatment for lack of appetite, wasting, weak blood, sluggish blood, all weaknesses of the arteries, heart disease, taken from one period to another it is reputed to aid conception in barren animals.

**Cats and Dogs -** A good female herb for abdominal ailments, injuries after delivery or damage and debility, to strengthen the developing foetus in the womb, for inclination to miscarry and prolapse of the uterus.

# Licorice

**Actions -** Demulcent, laxative, adrenal stimulant, expectorant, sialagogue.

The root part is used , possessing unique pectoral and emollient properties, it is also nutritive and slightly laxative, It contains the building blocks of hormones, has a marked effect on the endocrine system, catarrh, bronchitis, coughs, gastric and peptic ulcers, abdominal colic. Use for the treatment of cough, inflamed throat, pneumonia, pleurisy, all catarrhal conditions, gallstones, chronic constipation, mild worms in young animals, female infertility, pains of colic.

# Marshmallow

**Actions -** Demulcent, diuretic, emollient, vulnerary.

The foliage of the mallow is eaten by all animals, the roots are the main part used in internal medicine and also the leaves which are especially used for inflammation of the stomach and bowel, it contains over half its weight in sweet tasting mucilage which possess unique properties of lubricating, soothing and healing. A poultice can be used for all inflammatory conditions. Use for the treatment of sore throats, pulmonary catarrhs, pleurisy, diarrhea, dysentery, bowel inflammations and haemorrhages.

# Mistletoe

**Actions** - Nervine, hypotensive, cardiac depressant, nervous tachycardia.

A tea is given in cases of chronic cramps, frostbite, hardening of the arteries, stroke, bleeding of the lungs and intestines, disorders of the uterus especially bleeding, is good as a general blood stauncher.

# Nettles

**Actions -** Astringent, tonic, diuretic.

Used to treat rheumatism, arthritis, defective circulation and it also can relieve depression, bronchitis and reduces the risk of haemorrhage. It is perhaps the best blood herb which it purifies and renews. It cleanses the stomach and circulatory system ridding the body of eczema and other chronic skin disorders. Tonic for the pancreas and cleans the urinary system.

# Parsley

**Actions** - Diuretic, carminative, emmenagogue, expectorant.

Well-liked by sheep and goats, improves their milk yield and keeps them free from foot ills. It is a great enricher of the blood being very rich in iron and copper. Nutrient, digestive tract tonic, diuretic, high in potassium minerals and vitamins, bladder and kidney infections, incontinence, blood cleanser, immune builder, tonic for the blood vessels, aids in afterbirth pains, mainly used as a diuretic, carminative and emmenagogue. Good for the treatment of all disorders of the kidneys and bladder, gravel, stones, congestion, cystitis, jaundice, obesity, dropsy, worms, rheumatism, sciatica, swellings of the joints, the root can be used for constipation and obstructions of the intestines. For any Animals that are recovering from an illness, surgery or toxic kidney problems. Can also add finely chopped parsley into their daily meals once or twice a week to help keep kidneys cleansed and free of disease.


## Plantain

**Actions** - Expectorant, demulcent, astringent, diuretic.

Goats and sheep enjoy its foliage and poultry seek out the seeds. Plantain clears heat and removes excess fluid from the body while at the same time soothing inflammation and irritated tissues. The whole plant yields soothing mucilage similar to linseed, gentle expectorant while soothing sore and inflamed membranes, coughs, bronchitis etc. Its astringency aids in diarrhea and cystitis where there is bleeding. Is good for using in the treatment of stomach ulcers and has been used for blood poisoning. The plant is high in chlorophyll and good for use on wounds.

**Uses** - Treatment of dysentery, hemorrhages, internal obstructions and ulcers, fevers.

**Externally** - Wounds, sores, ulcers and all bites, eye disorders.

**Cats and Dogs -** Plantain is used for the entire range of diseases of the respiratory organs, particularly congested lungs, bronchial asthma and TB. It purifies the blood, lungs and stomach and is good for bad blood, kidney disorders, eczema, herpes and coughs. It helps convalescents especially when they need to gain weight. Also used in liver and bladder diseases.


## Rosemary

**Actions -** Circulatory and nerve stimulant, carminative, antispasmodic, antidepressive.

The powdered form is used on wounds as a antiseptic, nerve tonic, carminative, insecticide, acts as a circulatory and nerve stimulant, headache. Used in the treatment of all ailments of the heart, rheumatism, fits, epilepsy, paralysis, gastritis, diarrhea, dysentery.

## Sage

**Actions -** Carminative, antispasmodic, astringent, antiseptic.

Sage is well liked by animals and as with other aromatics makes the milk refreshing, tonic and increases the milk yield, it is a nervine, digestive and blood cleanser, a first rate remedy for all disorders of the throat, lungs and ears, inflamed and bleeding gums, inflamed tongue or general mouth inflammation, mouth ulcers, a good mouth wash.

**Uses -** Treatment of nerve debility, paralysis, all gastric ailments, constipation, obesity and female ailments, eczema, fevers, wound infections.

**Caution -** Stimulates the muscles of the uterus so should be avoided during pregnancy.

**Cats and Dogs -** For inflammations of the mout , throat and tonsils.

## Shepherds Purse

**Actions -** Uterine stimulant, astringent, diuretic.

Possesses important astringent properties, all animals like this herb and poultry seek it eagerly.

A gentle diuretic, diarrhea, wounds, reduces excessive menstruation.

**Uses -** Treatment of haemorrhages internal and external, profuse bleeding of deep wounds, kidney ailments, female problems.

Cats and Dogs - For all internal and external bleeding tisanes should be given, helpful in muscular complaints and muscular atrophy.

## Slippery Elm

**Actions -** Demulcent, astringent, nutrient.

Slippery elm bark provides a nutritious gruel which also possesses remarkable medicinal properties acting as a poultice both internally and externally. A nutrient and food for very old or young or weak cats and dogs, coats and heals all inflamed tissues internally and externally and is used for the stomach, intestines, ulcers, ulcerative colitis, enteritis, dysentery, constipation, internal bleeding of the digestive tract. Use for treatment of all digestive complaints especially ulcers for which it is a specific, dysentery, all pectoral disorders including TB, lung and bronchial hemorrhage, wasting diseases, rickets, stunted growth.

# Speedwell

**Actions -** Expectorant, diuretic, stomachic, tonic.

Has a strong purifying action and will clear bronchitis, digestive disorders and asthma. It is also effective in the treatment of sores, eczema and ulcers especially when they are of the moist weeping kind. It rids the intestines of mucous and unhealthy deposits and can also be used for liver and spleen disorders.

# St John's Wort

**Actions** - Anti-inflammatory, astringent, sedative, nervine, anti-viral, nerve pains, anti-spasmodic, vulnerary, antibacterial.

The name St John's Wort came from the Knights of St John of Jerusalem who used the herb to treat battle wounds.

**Uses** - Taken internally has a sedative and pain reducing effect, neuralgic pain, anxiety, tension, rheumatic pain, sciatica, for pains that shoot along the nerves, as a lotion it will speed the healing of wounds and bruises and is used where there is damage to the nerve rich areas, varicose veins and mild burns. Good for inflamed joints and rheumatic pain. In humans recently the herb has become popular to use as a antidepressant especially for cases of anxiety. Use as a lotion on wounds especially in the nerve rich areas such as the lips and fingers. As a lotion it is commonly mixed with Calendula, Homoeopaths call this lotion Hypercal.

**Caution** - Animals that overdose on Hypericum especially cattle become photosensitive and have to be locked in the barn for a while so as not to become sun burnt.

**Cats and Dogs** - Excellent wound herb and good for all nerve injuries. Good for highly strung, hysterical cats and dogs or those who have suffered some emotional or physical trauma.

# Thyme

**Actions** - Carminative, antimicrobial, antispasmodic, astringent, expectorant, anthelmintic.

Used for laryngitis, sore throat and tonsils as well as being good for digestive infections and problems.

# Valerian

**Actions** - Sedative, antispasmodic, carminative, anxiety, antidepressive, hypotensive.

A powerful nervine and sedative stronger than other herbal sedatives, pain reliever, reduces anxiety, hysteria, sooths the nervous system, reduces high blood pressure, slows and strengthens the heart and calms palpitations, useful for muscle spasm, arthritic pain, spinal injuries, aids indigestion and gas, insomnia, cramps, colic, can help with migraines. Used for the treatment of epilepsy, hysteria, acute constipation, worms, malaria, pain, sensitive nervous animals.

# Yarrow

**Actions** - Diuretic, antiseptic, diaphoretic, peripheral vaso dilator, hypotensive, bitter tonic. All abdominal complaints even cancer. When the queen suffers from inflammation of the ovaries or prolapse of the uterus, for feline respiratory disease to relieve congestion and running eyes. Bone marrow problems and diseases, bleeding from the lungs and stomach, good for flatulence, indigestion and abdominal cramps, soothes the gastro intestinal tract and calms diarrhoea. Gives the kidneys a boost. Good for fevers.

# Witch Hazel

**Actions** - Astringent one of the most widely used ones. Antiseptic.

As with all astringents this herb may be used where ever there is bleeding both externally and internally, commonly used for piles, bruises and inflamed swellings, varicose veins, diarrhea.

Use internally to heal ulcerated and burnt tissues in cases of poisoning, stomach and intestinal ulcers, Externally - wounds, sores, bruises, ulcers, inflammation of the organs of reproduction, torn udders resulting in milk leakage, inflamed udders and glands, sore eyes and inflamed ears.

# Homeopathic Supplement

Homeopathy has been around now for hundreds of years and unlike most other forms of medicine its rules have not changed and will not for they are based on a essential truth. The main rule is Like cures Like or if we break down the word Homeopathy homo means the same and pathy means disease. As Homoeopathy is a very hard science to learn and as it kind of sits or balances on the border of hard science and metaphysics I will not try to explain to you what it is here as it would probably take a whole book to do this but I will say this, in the UK and a lot of countries in Europe it is on and paid for by the National Health System and anything that can get a politician to open their purse must work. It is said that Homeopathy sits on a three legged stool. What this means is that if a remedy has at least three symptoms in the same strength as the symptoms you are trying to match then that remedy is a potential cure for your condition or if not cure it will offer the condition relief. The more symptoms you can match to the remedy the better the remedy will work for the rule is likes cure likes not vaguely similar cures. Listed below are some common Homoeopathic Remedies and some of the symptoms they cover. The idea is to find one remedy that covers most of your symptoms. To make the remedies as closer a match as we can we ask lots of questions like the ones below and after we gather all the answers we have what is called a good Symptom Picture which we then try to match as accurately as we can to a Remedy. Most Homeopathic Materia Medicas are set out to answer the questions listed below with the mind symptoms being the most important. Questions on time, position and temperature are good for making a choice between to very close remedies. The best Materia Medica for the lay person is Boerickes and you should be able to view this on a few Homeopathic websites.

# Symptom Guide Questions

1. Was there a sudden onset of the condition, at what time?
2. What time of the day does the patient feel either better or worse.
3. What is the effect of motion? jarring? walking? running?
4. What is the effect of drinking fluids? warm and or cold drinks?
5. Is the patient thirsty or not at all? sips or gulps?
6. Is the onset from exertion? overeating? weather changes? emotions?
7. Mental emotional state of patient?
8. Better warm room? warm air?
9. Better cool room? cool open air?
10 Are the respirations upper chest movements or in the abdomen?
11 Respirations - dry or wet?
12 Expectoration - watery or stringy mucous, easy or difficult.
13 Is there coughing
14 Position - better or worse from sitting? standing? lying? lying on which side?
15 Along with the condition is there fever? gas? belching? wind?

**Modality** - The questions above are covering what the Homoeopaths call modalities which basically mean are covering a condition that makes the patient better or worse. I will list the main Modalities below. The Modalities help us to distinguish which remedy is right for the case especially when we have a group that look as though they may all work which is what I am giving you und the disease heading. Using modalities forces you to think what really is going on, is this the nature of the beast or the nature of the disease.

**Time** - Better or Worse morning, night, weekly, monthly, seasonally etc.

**Motion** - Better or Worse first movement, rest, exertion, walking, stretching, rising up etc

**Temperature** - Better or Worse heat, cold, cold air blowing, sudden change etc.

**Body Activity** - Better or Worse eating, drinking, urinating, defecating, sleep, coughing etc

**Weather** - Better or Worse, damp, sunny, foggy, storms, sudden changes etc.

**Senses** - Better or Worse - touch, pressure, noise, light, odours etc.

**Position** - Better or Worse lying, standing, sitting, stretched out, doubled up, right side etc.

**Mind** - Excitement, anger, fear, stress, better busy, nervous all the time etc.

Now read through all the remedies in the Marteria Medica (Homoeopathic Remedy Reference) and you will notice that most of them have Mind or mental symptoms kind of describing the personalities or moods a good example is Nux Vomica, I think we all know a nasty type of individual that this remedy would be suited to and meaning as though the individual is suited to this remedy then the remedy would have a curative action on them but don't expect it to change the nature of the beast. One of the main rules of Homeopathy is the closer the match of the remedy the higher the Potency you use but if you are not used to Homoeopathy just use the 30C potency and remember what I said about the 3 legged stool. Potency is a measure of strength and depth of action.

Remember as mentioned before Homoeopathy sits on a three legged stool. What this means is that if a remedy has at least three symptoms in the same strength as your symptoms then that remedy is a potential cure.

**Note -** The best prescribing guide for the layman is **Boerickes Materia Medica With Repertory.**

Another good guide is **The Complete Book of Homeopathy by Dr Michael Weiner.**

I always buy my books on Homeopathy from India as they are quarter the price and there is always a wide selection. Put B. Jain Publishers into the google search engine go to their web site and check out these books and I am sure you will be pleased with what you find.

# Disease Nosodes

Nosodes are remedies made from disease material mainly from the tissues, discharges, exudates, excretions, suppurations or secretions of a infected being. Simply stated a Nosode is a homeopathic remedy prepared from a pathological specimen. Rabies Nosode, for example starts with the saliva of a rabid dog and is then potentized.

Nosodes have many uses and are widely used in homeopathic practice to help limit cases of infectious diseases and to help during the recovery phase of a disease especially the ones that linger and drag on. There are Nosodes for most infectious diseases of animals and humans the use of Nosodes in this way is referred to as isopathy rather than Homoeopathy. They are often used in farm situations, to limit the spread and the effects of infectious diseases. This has especially been used as a vital component of mastitis control on many farms, both organic and conventional. One documented event about Nosodes dates back to Napoleon marching his Legions through Europe and spreading Typhoid in their wake, the towns that had the best cure rates were the ones where the local Homoeopaths used a Nosode of the disease.

Nosodes can be used in the prevention of infectious diseases in the manner of vaccination but they work by a completely different mechanism then from the raising of antibodies that vaccines work by. As yet it is not actually known how they work but they have survived hundreds of years ridicule by producing results and will carry on doing so.

The best known study into Nosodes was done by Dr. Christopher Day of England involving 'kennel cough' in a boarding kennel. At the time he was called in, there were 40 dogs in the kennel with 35 that had kennel cough. About half had been vaccinated for this malady. He gave a Nosode to all the animals that were there and all the dogs that came in through the rest of the summer, which was another 214 dogs. He successfully reduced the incidence of kennel cough from over 90% to less than 2%.

Nosodes used for the prevention of diseases are usually given in the 30C potency. A good dosing regime is one dose given night and morning for 3 days followed by one per month for the next 6 months.

This generally provides a good level of protection after the first week. A good example of how this can be used is a puppy given the Nosode of Parvovirus at 3 to 4 weeks of age instead of having to wait for 9 weeks for the vaccination, this way the puppy is protected before given the vaccination.

Nosodes can have homeopathic therapeutic properties in their own right. Such Nosodes are found in the Homoeopathic Materia Medica and have undergone a proper 'proving'. Examples are Bacillinum, Carcinosinum, Medorrhinum, Psorinum, Tuberculinum.

**Dose -** Dr. Surjit S. Makker recommends 20ml of remedy mixed with 8 liters of water for 100 birds. This medicated water should be shaken well and put in drinkers accordingly. For individual birds give them 2-3 pellets by mouth and keep them calm.

# Materia Medica

**Note - All Homeopathic Remedies are given in Potency and not in material Form.**

# Aconite

**Characteristics -** Aconite is best used in the first stages of a illness, especially when fear and anxiety are present. Symptoms appear suddenly, without warning and they may be caused by exposure to cold winds or draughts or by a severe fright. Symptoms are a marked restlessness, animal displays extreme anxiety or fear, high fever with a burning skin, extreme sweating and a burning thirst, a hoarse dry painful cough, bright light noises stress and cold worsen the symptoms, rest and quiet relieves the symptoms. The pains of Aconite are unbearable, sharp, shooting, burning pains, tingling and numbness. A remedy for fevers and inflammatory states, use at the first sign of all fevers, shivering with cold sweats, difficult breathing, animal shows desire for large quantities of water, symptoms worse at midnight, symptoms improve in the open air.

**Mind -** Great fear, anxiety, restlessness, extreme sensitivity to pain, worry, foreboding.

**Better** - In open air, warmth, rest.

**Worse** - In the evening and night, particularly before midnight, lying on affected side.


## Allium Cepa

**Characteristics** - Increased secretions from the eyes and nose, like those of the common cold. Frequent sneezing with watery discharge which burns the nose and upper lip, but the eye discharge is bland and doesn't burn (the opposite of Euphrasia). Tickling in the throat with incessant cough (feels as if larynx is split) holds throat when coughing. Being in cool open air relieves the symptoms, eyelids are swollen and red, abdominal tympany with wind, this remedy is indicated in the early stages of most catarrhal conditions, mild forms of cat flu can be cut short if given early.

**Better** - Cold room (except cough), open air.

**Worse** - Evening, warm room, odours.


## Antimonium Tartaricum - Ant Tart

**Characteristics** - Is characterized by a loose rattling unproductive cough such as is often herd in cats. Respiration can be very difficult with much gasping. There is usually thirst for little and often. Symptoms are worse in the evening, lying down and in cold damp weather or a warm room. Confined largely to respiratory diseases, abundant bronchial secretions, great rattling of mucous with little expectoration, drowsiness, debility and sweat.

**Mind** - Drowsy and despondent, fear of being alone, child will not be touched without whining.

**Better** - Sitting erect, from burping and expectoration.

**Worse** - Evenings, lying down, damp cold weather.


## Apis

**Characteristics** - Apis is used for various types of swelling and inflammation such as that from animal bites and bites and stings from insects, it is also used for measles, mumps, sore throats, sore red eyes and fever. Apis is a quick acting remedy for inflammations especially those ones with edema and lots of swelling which is its main use.  Acute nephritis with scanty and burning urine there may be some blood in the urine. . Symptoms are swelling with edema which makes the effected parts look shiny, red and puffy, the swollen parts feel soggy and waterlogged, a fever that develops rapidly but without thirst, extreme restlessness and fidgeting, an irritable nature and perhaps jealous, cool air and cold compresses relieve the symptoms. Pains are burning and stinging, arthritis with swelling, animals seek cold surface to lie on, swollen eyelids, may be swollen ears, may be blood in the urine, in the horse and cow there may be edema in the lower limbs while in dogs abdominal dropsy is seen. Symptoms get worse from heat and improve in the open air and from cold bathing.

**Mind** - Apathy, indifference, awkward.

**Better** - By cold, (room, air or application)

**Worse** - From warmth, pressure, late in the afternoon, from sleeping.

## Arnica

**Characteristics** - Bruises and similar injuries where the skin is unbroken and there is mental or emotional shock. Symptoms are any type of bruising or similar injury caused by crushing, squeezing or wrenching, muscles strains which feel sore and bruised, shock after accidents, there is a fear of being touched because of the pain, good for the soreness after birth and medical operations.

Arnica can be used in potency and also as a cream. The cream must not be used on broken skin or wounds. Animal shrinks away when you try to touch it, symptoms improve when lying down.

**Mind** - Fears touch or approach, whole body oversensitive.

**Better** - Lying down or with head low.

**Worse** - Least touch, motion, damp and cold.

# Arsenic Album

**Characteristics** - Burning pains relieved by heat, anxious, restless, weak and chilly with an air of fear and hopelessness. Anxiety or restlessness are often present where this remedy is indicated. Discharge from eyes and nose are watery and acrid causing ulceration in those regions. The mouth is usually dry and the patient is usually thirsty. Dramatic vomiting and diarrhea often simultaneously indicate its use if the modalities agree. The patient may have wheezing respiration and allergic asthmatic conditions can respond well. The skin can be dry, scaly and scruffy. Symptoms are worse for cold and wet better for warmth. Tries to find relief in motion but immediately feels weak with movement. Restless, feels cold, complains of general weakness, discharges burn the skin.

**Mind** - Fear with despair and restlessness.

**Better** - Warmth, open air, relieved by sweat, hot drinks, lying down (but restless).

**Worse** - Cold air, after midnight eg 1 to 3am. Wet damp weather and near sea shore.


# Belladonna

**Characteristics -** This is one of the great fever remedies, conditions requiring its use usually being of violent and sudden onset. Heat, redness, pain and swelling characterize its symptoms. It is one of the main remedies used in convulsions. Pupils are usually dilated which is a keynote for this remedy. Acute ear inflammation where there is heat, pain and swelling, respond well. The mouth is usually dry and there is great thirst. With Belladonna always think BIRDS. B for burning, I for irritability, R for redness, D for delirium and S for spasms.

**Mind** - Hallucinations, delirium, rages, bites, strikes, desire to escape.

**Better -** For quiet, dark, rest with slight warmth.

**Worse -** For noise, touch or jarring motion.

# Bellis Perennis

**Characteristics** - Trauma to abdomen and pelvic organs especially after surgery and child birth if arnica does not give relief. Injuries to the nerves with intense soreness, back ache from hard physical work such as gardening, pain is bruised sore and aching, better cold presses, worse touch, after getting wet.

The animal is unwilling to move and when made to do so evinces pain, muscular stiffness is prominent.

**Worse** - Left side and cold wind.

# Bryonia

**Characteristics** - This remedy shows both diarrhea and constipation symptoms, the latter usually in chronic conditions. The mouth is often dry and there is great thirst. The tongue is often coated yellow. It is of great help in many cases of rheumatism or arthritis where the symptoms agree. There is often respiratory signs with a hoarse hacking cough. All symptoms are worse for movement and better for rest.

**Mind** - Irritable, delirium.

**Better** - Lying on the painful side, pressure, rest and cold things.

**Worse** - Warmth, motion, morning, eating and touch.

# Calendula

**Characteristics** - The part used is the Flowers and it is used for wounds and skin irritations, it is healing, soothing, anti-inflammatory, astringent, anti-fungal and anti-microbial.

Use as a lotion for cuts, grazes, infected sores, fungal infections, any skin inflammations, regulates the oil production of the skin so is good for acne, to stop bleeding, for bruises and sprains, skin ulcers and minor burns and scolds.

**Note** - The tincture of this is used as a lotion diluted at 1 to 10.

# Cantharis

**Characteristics -** Important first aid remedy for minor burns and for other pains that feel burning and fiery, also has a healing effect on the bladder, urethra and other parts of the urinary tract where burning pain is the key symptom, burns and scalds especially where blistering and inflammation occur, sunburn, insect bites that feel hot and burn, cystitis. Pains are violent burning, cutting, stabbing or smarting, rawness, use when the animal appears distressed when passing urine, or tries to pass and cannot. Better from warmth rest and rubbing.

**Mind** - Furious delirium, acute mania generally of a sexual type, crying, barking.

**Better** - From rubbing

**Worse** - From touch or approach, from urinating, from drinking cold water.

# Carbo Vegetabilis

**Characteristics -** Patient exhibits mental and physical sluggishness and symptoms come on slowly, generalized weakness of all functions especially digestion, overweight, torpid, lazy, complaints of coldness, pains usually described as burning, pressing pains, wishes to be fanned, digestive problems such as belching often accompany any illness.

**Mind -** Aversion to darkness, sudden loss of memory.

**Better** - Being fanned, passing gas, rest.

**Worse** - Morning and evening, exertion, cold, tight clothes at abdomen.

# Causticum

**Characteristics -** Burns and burning pains such as cystitis also used for dry coughs, burns to the skin especially with marked inflammation and blistering, coughs, laryngitis and hoarseness from straining and over using voice, cystitis especially with involuntary passing of urine when coughing, chronic cystitis, exposure to cold dry air may make symptoms worse.

**Mind** - Least thing makes it cry, sad, hopeless. Ailments from long lasting grief.

**Better** - In damp wet weather, warmth.

**Worse** - Cold winds.

## Euphrasia

**Characteristics -** Affects the mucous membranes of the eyes, nose and chest producing copious watery secretions, eye secretions cause smarting of the skin while the nose discharge is bland. Used for conjunctivitis, eye strain generally  but especially from computers, eyes that feel sore and inflamed and look red, hay fever symptoms including a tickly throat, sneezing, a runny nose, and itchy red watering eyes. Sunlight wind and warmth worsen the symptoms. Use for Dogs who have had their head out of the window for too long, symptoms better in dim light or darkness, in all species a tendency to diarrhea occurs.

**Better** - In the dark

**Worse** - From light, indoors, in the evening.

## Hypericum

**Characteristics -** Used for bruises and other injuries especially to nerve rich areas like the fingers, lips, ears, eyes ,tail bone, good for the pain of puncture wounds of any cause e.g. animal or insect. Helps with the pains after operations especially amputations. Pains are violent shooting pains along a nerve path, burning, tingling and numbness. Worse from shock and touch and better from rubbing, horse fly bites, symptoms worse cold better warmth.

**Mind** - Anxiety, melancholy, effects of shock.

**Better** - Bending head backward.

**Worse** - Cold, dampness and touch.

# Ipecac

**Characteristics -** Indicated for complaints of persistent nausea not relieved by vomiting, ailments caused by eating rich or indigestible type of foods such as ice-cream, sweets etc., useful to stop bleeding if blood is bright red.

**Mind -** Easily irritated, child cries or screams continuously, wanting something but not sure what they desire, holds everything in contempt.

**Worse -** Warm, moist weather, lying down.

# Kali Bichromicum

**Characteristics -** Has a affinity for the mucous membranes of the body, tough stringy viscid secretions sometimes forming thick yellow green mucous, sinus infections, suited for fleshy fat light complexioned people, general weakness.

**Better -** Heat

**Worse -** Cold, beer, morning, undressing.

# Kali Carbonicum

**Characteristics -** Has a affinity for the mucous membranes digestive and respiratory, very tired, anaemic, flabby tissues which may be swollen, sweat, backache, weakness, many conditions have a aggravation at 2am to 4am, often stays immobile when ill.

**Mind -** Very irritable, hypersensitive to pain, despondent.

**Better -** During the day, sitting down, bending forward, warmth.

**Worse -** Cold weather, between 2am and 4am.

# Lachesis

**Characteristics -** Many symptoms tend to be left sided, cannot bear tight clothing, symptoms worse on awakening, symptoms relieved with onset of the menstrual flow. Short dry cough, feels relief after coughing up watery phlegm, feeling of constriction in throat and chest, better bending forward.

**Mind -** Overly talkative, impatient, sad, jealous, no desire to mix with world.

**Better -** Release of pressure, eating fruit, cold, discharges.

**Worse -** Pressure, touch, after sleep, heat, hot weather.


# Ledum

**Characteristics -** Has a action on the capillaries and is useful for cleaning up bruises especially around the eyes, mainly used for puncture wounds made by sharp points such as nails and wood splinters and insect bites and stings especially ones that don't heal properly and look blue and puffy. Wounds that feel cold to the touch, septic conditions, sprains, pains are throbbing, tearing, prickling, they shoot upwards, stiff and sore. Better cold, cold bathing. This remedy was used in the past along with hypericum to ward off tetanus especially in deep wounds

**Better -** From cold.

**Worse -** At night and from heat.


# Lycopodium

**Characteristics -** Exerts most of its effects on the digestive organs, liver, kidneys and respiratory systems. The patient dislikes being left alone and appears apprehensive. The nose is often blocked and there may be blisters on the tongue. Eating a little food always satisfies the appetite but appetite is very marked. The belly is usually bloated. The stool appears hard and small and is expelled only with difficulty accompanied by ineffectual straining. Urination is also a slow process and the urine has a red sediment. Symptoms are worse for heat generally and better for cold.

**Mind -** Melancholy, afraid to be alone, apprehensive.

**Better -** By motion, on getting cold.

**Worse -** From heat.

# Natrum Sulphuricum

**Characteristics** - A good liver remedy, emotional and mental difficulties arising after head injury, useful in problems associated with rainy weather and dampness, patient feels every change from dry to wet weather, may remove excess water and fluid retention from the body.

**Mind** - Lively music saddens, melancholy, inability to think, dislikes to speak or be spoken to.

**Better** - Dry weather and environments, pressure, change of position.

**Worse** - Damp weather, damp basements, lying on left side.


# Nux Vom

**Characteristics** - The remedy for overindulgence, adapted especially to thin irritable energetic people who attend with great detail to tasks, quarrelsome, nervous, intelligent, hypochondriacal, oversensitive to noise music and light, craves stimulants.

Primarily used in the digestive sphere, its greatest reputation is in helping disturbances following overeating of unsuitable foods. Feces is usually hard but diarrhea can follow overeating. There is abdominal discomfort, flatulence, irritability and sensitivity to noise. Symptoms are generally worse for noise and better after rest or for damp weather.

**Mind** - Very irritable, sensitive to all impressions, malicious, disposed to reproach others.

**Better** - Wet weather, lying down, uninterrupted nap.

**Worse** - Overeating, mental over exertion, sensory stimulation ie sound, sight, touch etc.


# Phosphorus

**Characteristics** - Irritated and inflamed mucous and serous membranes are the key feature of this remedy. Is a very sudden remedy with suddenness of symptoms. The patient is sensitive to loud and sudden noises (eg thunder fireworks etc). Degenerative processes and bone destruction respond well to Phosphorus. Food is suddenly vomited back up when it has been warmed in the stomach, gums can be ulcerated and bloody. Hepatitis, jaundice, pancreatic disease and nephritis come into its sphere. Urine may be bloody. A very painful cough is also a symptom. Wounds that perpetually bleed may also be helped. The patient is usually in poor body condition. Symptoms are worse for touch, exertion, in the evening and during thunder storm. Better for cold and sleep.

**Mind** - Low spirits, restless, fidgety.

**Better** - In the dark, lying on the right side, from the cold, sleep.

**Worse** - Touch, from exertion and in the evening.


# Pulsatilla

**Characteristics -** Often indicated for those with mild, gentle, timid yielding dispositions who are easily moved to laughter and tears, The Pulsatilla person wants to be held and loved, moods changeable and fickle, the patient is chilly but desires strolling in cold air, symptoms are erratic and change frequently, pains are wandering, pains that grow gradually in intensity, fever without thirst despite dry mouth, bland yellow discharges.

**Mind -** Weeps easily, timid, fears to be alone - dark - ghosts, likes sympathy and fuss, highly emotional, easily discouraged, sensitive.

**Better -** Open air, cold applications, consolation relieves symptoms.

**Worse -** Evening before midnight, warmth, after eating fat rich food.


# Rhus Tox

**Characteristics -** Is the most famous of the rheumatic remedies. The skin and muscular skeletal system are its main spheres. Small red papules in the skin and sometimes vesicles are typical lesions with much scratching. In all cases of damage to muscles think of Rhus and the symptoms of arthritis which are worse after rest particularly if this follows strenuous exertion. The symptoms improve with limbering up, The worst pains are seen as the animal arises from its bed.

**Mind** - Listless, sad, extreme restlessness, great apprehension at night.

**Better** - Warmth, walking, from stretching out limbs.

**Worse** - During sleep, cold wet rainy weather and at night.

## Ruta

**Characteristics** - Has effects on the joints, tendons, cartilages, and the periosteum which is a fine membrane that covers bones and gives it that shiny look, it is also used for eye strain where the vision goes dim.

Used for painful bruises affecting the bones, dislocations, strains to the tendons or joints, aching with restlessness, pains are gnawing, digging, burning, bruised, sore as if beaten, bones as if broken, pain deep in the bones, rheumatism.

**Better** - From lying and warmth.

**Worse** - From over exertion, touch, cold wet weather.

## Silica

**Characteristics** - Fits the shy chilly patient who is reluctant to enter the room, chronic inflammatory conditions such as sinus, helps in the removal of foreign bodies such as splinters and seeds, ripens abscesses, ailments attended with pus formation. Use silica and be prepared to use it for a while sometimes up to 3 weeks.

**Mind** - Faint hearted, anxious, yielding.

**Better** - Warmth, wet or humid weather.

**Worse** - Morning, from lying down, cold.

## Staphysagria

**Characteristics** - Suits sensitive people who suppress their feelings and suffer in silence or who boil over with indignation, remedy for cuts and wounds especially those that are from medical procedures and have the mentioned feelings. Nervous states of animals. The pains are stinging, stitching, smarting, squeezing, as if stabbed by a knife. Worse from touch, emotions and suppressed anger.

**Better** - Warmth, rest at night.

**Worse** - Touch on affected parts, loss of fluids.

## Symphytum

**Characteristics -** Causes bone to grow and promotes fast healing should be given for all fractures. Used for injuries to the hard parts of the body while arnica is for the soft parts. Also used for eye injuries caused from blows.

**Caution** - Do not use if a pin has been placed in the bone as the pin has to be removed latter.

## Tarentula Cubensis

**Characteristics -** For abscesses, boils, carbuncles, swellings of any kind but especially on the back of the neck where the skin turns black, red/blue or purple with great pain. Deep septic conditions with hardening of the effected part, condition comes on fast, pains are burning, stinging, throbbing, pricking like a needle.

**Worse** - Night.

## Urtica Urens

**Characteristics -** Can be used for burns and also for cystitis where the urine burns the skin and there is difficulty passing urine. Symptoms are stinging pains, swellings particularly blistery swellings, itching.

**Worse** - Cool moist air, touch.

# Vitamin C

Vitamin C is the primary antioxidant in the lungs and a powerful antihistamine without side effects. Low vitamin C dramatically increases histamine levels which put you at greater risks for inflammation responses in the body. Always give a high dose of Vitamin C to animals before any operation where they require a anaesthetic for the reasons mentioned above as they will recover faster and better from the anaesthetic and maybe the inflammation from the surgical incisions will be toned down a bit.

Vitamin C is needed by the immune system and is necessary for healing and the prevention of infections along with being a potent antioxidant with anti-bacterial and antiviral actions. It is also essential for the utilization of the essential amino acids lysine (anti-viral) and proline. Another point to consider is that stress depletes the bodies supply of Vitamin C so this may be another factor in the cause of many diseases. Vit C is essential for the formation of collagen tissue which is vital in tendons and cartilage so always consider this in muscle and back injuries and especially trauma injuries.

Sodium Ascorbate is good for use on animals as it is virtually tasteless when added to the animal's food and does not curdle milk. This can be used in high doses when needed for example dose till the bowels become loose then back the dose off. For severe situations you can use a injectable Vitamin C, in Australia we use Troys Injectable Vit C which we get from the Agricultural Stock Feed Shops or Co Ops. Use a large gauge needle with this as some animals have rather thick hides and the liquid solution is also fairly thick.

Think of using Vitamin C in all operations and all acute diseases. It is a good last resort to think of before the rifle especially in the deadly acute diseases where as a last resort you would use the injectable form in a intramuscular injection, this can also be a good gauge as to what may happen as these injections hurt like hell so if the animal turns around and gives you a filthy look then there is a good chance that they may live and if they do not seem to notice the injection well the chances don't look too good. So remember always keep a bottle of Injectable C in the fridge for emergencies.

## Good Herb Sources of Vitamin C

Alfalfa, Burdock, Catnip, Cayenne, Chickweed, Dandelion, Hawthorn, Garlic, Horseradish, Kelp, Parsley, Plantain, Papaya, Raspberry, Rosehips, Shepherds Purse, Yellow Dock.

# Notes

# Global Warming Edition
## Fire, Heat Stress and Global Warming

As I am writing this during summer in the State of Victoria, Australia in the Countryside, the top of Australia in the Northern Territory has a fire burning which is the size of Spain. It just seems to be getting worse all the time. Australia is notorious for its massive fires and now the severity is getting worse, but luckily over a period of 20 years we have changed our habits and ways of thinking and quite a few times now we have managed to save ourselves when the Authorities were overwhelmed and could not help, or the roads were cut off so they couldn't get there anyway. Most farms big, small or Hobby Farms and even isolated properties now have trailers with a 1000 litre IBC tank hooked up to a pump and hose that can be transported where it is needed. Quite a few times now when the roads are blocked local communities have saved themselves with these trailers and on a lot of occasions some people call their friends for help and to bring their fire trailers over. With mobile phones they have now found that they can organize themselves and get multiple trailers out to deal with spot fires and have the situation under control before the Authorities get there. Now with the technical advancement and the falling of prices for drones you can even have a look at what is happening before you even get there or on your way. As far as I am concerned this is the way it should be and as the situation is only going to continue to get worse more people should start to prepare themselves for the worst. As the conditions get worse across the globe many people in remote areas are going to have to learn to look after themselves for as usual most of the help will go to the cities and large towns, so now is the time to start making your plans.

# High Temperature Animal Management Needs Good Planning

You need to develop a plan for days of high to extreme temperatures to ensure that your animals will have sufficient shade and water when needed in extreme weather conditions. Extreme heat causes significant stress for all animals with some suffering more than others, so now is the time to review your planning and farm infrastructure so as to provide shaded areas with good ventilation to maximise heat loss. As a gauge we will use 36 degrees Celsius as our danger mark especially if the heat is dry, if it is humid we can relax a bit, but it's time to get our act together. Managing animals in high temperatures requires good forward planning and keeping an eye on the weather forecasts along with developing a plan for days of high to extreme temperatures is essential in ensuring that your animals will have sufficient shade and water on those very hot days. More shade and water troughs would be a good start along with checking the animals more frequently during the hottest days at the hottest times of the day for signs of heat stress, along with all the water points to ensure animals have access to plenty of clean cool water. Make sure troughs or containers are firmly fixed so they cannot overturn and are clean, well designed and maintained to prevent injuries. Make sure the stock does not have to walk too far for water and that they know where all the water areas are and if you use large concrete troughs these will to help keep the drinking water cool. Extreme heat causes significant stress for all animals and it's up to you to ensure the welfare of your animals is maintained. Animals need to be checked regularly throughout the day for signs of heat stress. Remember with Global Warming there is no such thing as normal weather patterns anymore and it's going to get worse before it gets better, if it ever gets better, but that's up to our Governments and the rich elite of the world which makes it even more depressing.

# Heat Shelters for Animals

Animals need shelter during extended periods of extreme temperatures especially the very young or old and animals that are in poor condition or sick. Every farm is different but they are all going to get hit with Climate Change one way or another along with the country areas and their populations, so now is the time to have a good look around and consider improvements and see what there is that's going to give you problems in the future. Walk around the property and try to see what's going to cause you trouble in the middle of summer. Where do I need to put shade, are there any sheltered areas that you could use or fence off in an emergency and may add more trees and shade. Due to storms getting worse it may be time to have another good look at your high ground and figure out how you could use it in a flood and maybe how you could save the water by creating dams or ponds. About 30 years ago I was on a farm built on the side of a hill in the subtropics in Queensland that had a near hit by a cyclone. We had to wait a week before we could get into town, and even then we had to pile everyone onto a truck to get there as a car would have been washed away. Ten years later I was on a farm in South Australia 60 to 70 kilometres North of Adelaide during a drought and they stopped us from using the slasher on the back of the tractor, as when the slasher hit a rock the spark off the blade would cause a fire. To be honest I am glad my times nearly up as the future is not really looking all that bright and the reality is that it's up to you now to look after and protect you and yours with maybe a little help from your friends. Now let's have a good look at what's out there to keep your animals cool and healthy in the heat to come. **The best type of shelter during extreme heat should protect the animals from the sun and allow for the cooling effect of wind.** Don't forget to put some water close by. Pets and small animals should be moved to cool areas of the house or a shed.

1/. **Shade Sails** - My favourite and the easiest and cheapest to do is the Shade Sails. These are easy to set up and can be used as a large or small scale setup, or just in the places where you need them. The simplest is the sail on three posts. The best ways to use these are to find the areas on your property with a bit of natural shade and see how much you can increase it using a simple cheap sail with 3 posts. A good and natural spot to choose would be where a stream is in a valley where the animals would head to naturally or any other area in your land that has a natural shelter or one that could be made easily. On different farms I have noticed that animals tend to hang out in certain areas when they rest so this may be a good spot. Another advantage is that you can easily take the shade down for winter so it doesn't have to wear out fast. Shade sails are about the fastest, cheapest and easiest way to go and are a good first choice with fast results.

2/. **Trees and Shelter Belts** – Lots of farms have these; usually they are in an area where it was not worth the effort to get rid of them or too hard to access, or even a danger to the livestock. Maybe it's time these areas are re-examined again to see if they can be used fully or partly as a Heat Refuge. While you are doing this also consider where you could place new trees with large canopies that are fast growing and native to you area. Also consider placing one of these trees beside each water trough to slow down the evaporation rate. Shelterbelts or Hedges are a good idea and can be as big and complex as your imagination. Always have them crossing the farm going East to West so when the sun rises in the east the animals can use the shade on the west and the opposite in the afternoon, so that leaves us with only the mid-day sun to sort out. Always remember to leave regular gaps in the belts and hedges so animals can pass through them easily but also more importantly to allow a breeze to blow through the gaps to help cool the animals. Trees have a cooling effect due to absorption of heat by the leaves. Always check out the fodder trees that can be grown or even better are native to your area and always try to make everything multi-purpose. For those that are interested in this and want more information find yourself a Permaculture Manual as that will give you all the information you need along with plants you can use as stock feed and trees you can use as what they call Pioneer Plants, which you use to protect and fertilize the tree you want to grow which dies off latter after it has finished its work.

**3/. - Placement and Construction of Livestock Sheds** – Placement is the first and most important consideration especially for heat, but saying that if you live in a place where they have nasty cold winters and lots of snow you will have to decide between which is worse for you and plan accordingly. In winter the sun is low on the horizon so maybe think about making a sleeping and resting area on the longest wall of the structure so as to capture the most heat in winter, then in summer when the sun is above it will run along the roof. Aluminium or galvanised steel are ideal roofs for shelters, kennels, and chicken coops as these materials are very good at reflecting the radiative rays of the sun. Other common construction materials are corrugated iron, timber and shade cloth. You may want to consider having the structures east to west so in summer the sun runs across the roof and maybe insulate the east and west walls. **Outdoor poultry houses** should be positioned in shaded areas away from the sun and in a place where it can get good airflow. Use wide overhangs at the eaves and solid end walls so as to make as much shade as possible. Don't forget that an angled roof will reflect more heat at the hottest time of the day and leave you room for adding insulation in the future if things get worse. Place the nesting boxes in the coolest part of the structure or maybe back to back down the centre as this might be a better place for all the seasons. Again consider insulation on the east and west walls. With any farm construction it is always better to build slightly bigger then smaller as you don't want the risk of animals getting crushed, smothered or injured and always consider the entrance and door sizes as again it's better to make them bigger and avoid future problems.

## Heat Stress Tolerances for livestock

Animals at high risk of heat stress are the young, black and dark coloured animals and animals that have been housed and not usually out in the sun with fair skin such as pigs. As always the sun will make it worse for the sick and injured of all kinds and greatly increase the rate of water needed. Heat stress tolerances also vary between different species and different places where animals are farmed so we need to know what's happening in our own area, and how it is going to affect the livestock and what the future outlook may be, as there is no going back now. Your area may not be suitable anymore, or another breed of the same species might be happier in your area. Better to make the decisions sooner than later as it will be far cheaper in the long run. In Australia I was on a farm up North in the subtropics so we got Anglo-Nubian Goats who handled the temperature a lot better than us and most of the other animals and as an added bonus we found them to be highly intelligent. Next we will take a look at how heat stress affects our main animals.

## Handling Hot Days and Transport Animals

Try to do all the animal work in the cool of the mornings or the evenings. It is not good for you or the animals to work in extreme heat unless absolutely necessary or in an emergency such as a fire. Some of the farms I have worked on in very hot areas we worked from 6am to 10am and then 2pm to 6pm, which made life more bearably for both the human and the animals. For cattle research has shown that movement or handling during hot weather can increase their body temperature by 0.5 to 3.5° C. Increased body temperature or heat stress will cause losses in livestock and impact on their ability to function. Moving animals during cooler hours can decrease the impact of high temperatures, with a good example being a delay in milking by an hour or more in the evenings can result in an increase in production of up to 1.5 litres per day per cow. Transport of animals should be planned so that climatic extremes are avoided and animals are transported during the cooler hours of the day or at night. I know of an example that went really wrong when the driver was doing all the right things, he was carrying chickens from Adelaide to Melbourne which is a distance of 750 kilometres. He was carrying chickens in cages with water on a semi-trailer which they always tarped so as to keep the wind off the chickens, and always drove through the night so there would be no heat stress and always stopped at the half way point to check that everything was fine. In the last part of the trip the tarp ripped on the side close to the back on the trailer and the poor chickens there had to endure 110 Kph winds for a few hours resulting in about a quarter of them were very naked and not happy. Unfortunately the new owner was not very impressed and asked him what the hell did you do to them, which was about the same time as the drivers offsider burst out in hysterical laughter. This was just one of those things, the driver did everything right, he drove in the cool air of night, he only stopped once to check the load and that was just for 5 minutes. The general rules for transporting animals especially sheep and cattle in severe heat conditions are to use the safest and quickest roots, try to do it in one trip so the breeze through the truck keeps the animals cool. If it is necessary to stop, park the vehicle in the shade and at right angles to the wind direction to improve wind flow between animals during hot weather. Keep the duration of stops to a minimum to avoid the build-up of heat while the vehicle is stationary. In extreme heat reduce stocking densities by about 15% so as to encourage more breezes throughout the trailer to keep the animals cool. In some States and especially in the outback you have to have powerful rifles so if you have an accident you can humanly put down those animals that need it.

## Heat Stress Effects on Animals

The general signs of heat stress are panting, increased respiration rate, increased water intake, loss of appetite, listlessness or lethargy, increased salivation and in severe cases unconsciousness and the possibility of death. Here we will go through the different animals and see how they handle excessive heat and what we can do to prevent problems. If your animals are showing signs of heat stress you need to cool them down so start with taking them to the shade, with the best areas being were there is a breeze. To add to this you could use a water sprinkler capable of adding a fine misty spray to reduce the heat even further. Do not soak the animals, just a little bit of mist frequently. If animals are too stressed to move, pick them up and move them or provide shade where they are especially for the larger and heavier animals such as cattle. With cattle the easiest solution is to get the truck and use the truck to block the sun then provide water in 20 litre buckets (or whatever you have), encourage them to drink small amounts often as, a large amount may cause shock and death. After that try to find the biggest water mister bottle you can and spray just spray one of them and see how they handle it especially on the legs and feet, don't try to pour a bucket of cold water on them as the shock could be too much, but they may like a big wet towel put over them. **I have decided to start here with Humans because if you don't look after yourself and get it you are not going to be much use to your animals.**

## Humans and Heat Stress

If you are have to deal with heat stress in animals then it's time to learn how to treat Humans with the same condition, as you may be the next victim. This condition can sneak up on you without you realizing what is happening especially if the sun is directly on you head. Heat exhaustion is the beginning of the journey towards heat stroke. One of the fastest ways of getting there is wandering around in the sun on a hot sunny day of over 36 degrees Celsius without a hat on in the middle of a cloudless day. This means the sun is right above you and is beginning to cook your brain very fast. You can develop some really weird symptoms fast and need to get out of the sun. Unfortunately I went through this at about 21 and learned my lesson well. Now that the climate is hotter this is a lesson we should all learn especially for our children's sake as they are the ones that are vulnerable now. Start with your basic First Aid. A pre-warning of Heat Stress can be **Heat Cramps** which usually happen when you work outside in the heat and are sweating a lot and you've used up your excess fluid, so the body decides to tell you by starting to cramp.

**Signs of heat stress**

Excessive sweating and cold, pale, clammy skin.

Headache.

Dizziness and confusion.

Loss of appetite and feeling sick.

Nausea and or vomiting.

Cramps in the arms, legs and stomach.

Fast weak pulse.

Tiredness weakness.

Being thirsty.

Headache.

Fainting.

Decreased Urine Output.

Take this as your warning sign and get rehydrated and have a rest in a shady cool area. Heat cramps are the mildest form of heat related illness. They are painful muscle cramps and spasms caused by your body's loss of salt and fluid due to excessive sweating. Heat cramps can occur during or after intense exercise and can be a symptom of a more serious heat exhaustion. To relieve the cramps drink some water or even better a rehydration solution which should be in every first aid kit and rest in a shaded cooler area and finish the work in a cooler part of the day. Sometimes we can miss out on the cramps and slowly work our way to Heat Exhaustion without releasing till it is too late. Check all the symptoms and start treatment quickly so as to not make the condition worse. The best you can do is get the patient into a cool house with the air-conditioning running and offer them a long cool drink or even better one with a rehydration formula mixed into it and observe the patient and see what happens. Are they over dressed for the conditions? If so suggest to them that they are overdressed for the conditions. If you are worried that the condition is getting worse don't hesitate to call for an ambulance as the phone operators are usually highly trained and can go through the issues with you.

### Signs of Heatstroke

Hot, Red, Dry or Damp Skin.

Cessation of sweating.

Body temperature of 38C (104F) or higher.

Fast Strong Pulse.

Decreased urine output.

Rapid and shallow breathing.

Rapid heartbeat.

Elevated or lowered blood pressure.

Confusion and disorientation.

Can be nausea and Dizziness.

Can be seizure.

Fainting - often the first sign in the elderly.

Remove the person from the heat to a cool shady area, if serious especially in the old and young seek emergency help if available. Remove excessive clothing and take note of vital signs such as pulse and temperature and record them along with the worst symptoms. Cool the person with whatever means available but be careful not to shock them, again it's the young and old you have to be very careful with as a shock could be the last straw. Put in a cool tub of water or a cool shower, spray with a garden hose, sponge with cool water, fan while misting with cool water, or place ice packs or cold, wet towels on the person's head, neck, armpits and groin. Was the person just affected by the heat? Or were they working and exerting themselves in the heat? Is it humid weather? Have you been drinking alcohol (dehydration)? When was the last time you had a drink of water? Without a quick response to lower body temperature, heatstroke can cause your brain or other vital organs to swell, possibly resulting in permanent damage which is why this condition is an emergency situation so it is best to get as much information as you can get, especially of any medication they are taking and talk to the emergency services and see what they have to say.

## Homoeopathic Remedies For
## Heat Stress and Heat Stroke

Below are Homoeopathic Remedies that can be used for Heat Stress and Stroke. These remedies can be used by Humans and Animals. Instead of giving a higher dose when you consider the situation is getting worse it may be better to go to a higher Potency and see what happens. If the situation gets worse which can easily happen in this condition especially in the old and young and you require Ambulance or Medical Treatment, ensure they know the patient has taken Homoeopathic Remedies as the remedies may be masking some of the symptoms. The most important things you can do while waiting medical help is to keep the patient hydrated, cool, comfortable and in a positive mood knowing that help is on the way.

## Remedies Heat Exhaustion

**China 6C to 30C -** Feeling totally wiped out, drained with trembling. Very useful where there has been excessive sweating and severe dehydration is a factor.

**Natrum Carb 6C to 30C -** A remedy for sunstroke with a headache that feels like a weight on the head. The person may experience weakness and exhaustion and be sensitive to heat. Important Remedy for Sunstroke when the patient is susceptible to changes in temperature. Good for sensitive people who always seem to get headaches from being in the sun. Remedy for debility and exhaustion and headache caused by the sun. Also good for the chronic effects of sun-stroke. Patient may complain of tiredness and extreme weakness due to hot weather. In most cases, the complaints may get worse with a little exertion.

**Gelsemium 6C to 30C -** Useful for sunstroke with dizziness, heavy eyelids and a headache that starts at the back of the head and radiates forward. The person may feel weak and lethargic and experience trembling. Light headed, droopy, drowsy, thirstless despite the heat. Occasional chills running up and down the spine. Useful in sun-stroke where there is a high temperature with drowsiness and they may feel weak and lethargic and experience trembling, tendency to coma.

**Lachesis 6C to 30C -** A good remedy for sun-headaches or after being in the sun where there is faintness and dizziness. The key indicator is the person feels worse after a sleep or nap.

## Sun (heat) Stroke

**Belladonna 6C to 30C -** Indicated for sudden, intense symptoms of sunstroke, including high fever, throbbing headache, red face and dilated pupils. The person may be restless, delirious and sensitive to light and noise. Skin is flushed, hot and dry, rapid strong pulse, pupils are fixed and dilated. Headache that is better for dark, silence and rest. The headache can have violent shooting pains in the head which come and go suddenly making the patient cry out. Heat about the head with cold feet. Blood shot eyes and visible throbbing of the carotids. Use for Sunstroke with Congestion of the Head and Face. People needing Belladonna will experience a burning sensation on the face, a severe congestive headache and redness in the eyes. The patient may faint due to weakness. The skin feels hot, red, and dry, and the complaints may aggravate with the least movement.

**Gelsemium 6C to 30C -** Light headed, droopy, drowsy, thirstless despite the heat. Occasional chills running up and down the spine. Useful in sun-stroke where there is a high temperature with drowsiness or tendency to coma. In Sunstroke when patient feels dull and drowsy. In such cases, there is weakness along with trembling. The patient may feel dizzy and confused. Works well when there is vertigo with a blurring of vision. In most cases, the patient may feel better on lying down.

**Glonoine 6C to 30C -** Suitable for sunstroke with a severe headache, pulsating or bursting sensation in the head and a feeling of heat in the head. The person may have a flushed face, dilated pupils and experience dizziness or confusion. Throbbing, bursting headache with a hot face and sweaty skin. A great remedy for the effects of sunstroke and congestive headaches. Indicated when the patient has a severe, sudden headache with a throbbing sensation. The patient complains of heaviness in the head, and a feeling that the head is about to burst. In most cases, the pain in the head may get better after sleeping.

**Lachesis 6C to 30C -** Good remedy for sun-headaches or after being in the sun where there is faintness and dizziness. The key indicator is the person feels worse after a sleep or nap. Lachesis is an important remedy for a patient who gets a pale face and may even faint during

Sunstroke. Nausea and vomiting, along with a cutting and pressing headache, may also occur. The head is very sensitive to touch, and the headache may get worse with a change in weather.

## Other Remedies to Consider

**Bryonia 6C to 30C -** Severe Headache worse for even a slight movement. Remedy to think of when the person has an *intense unquenchable thirst for water.* The person is definitely better for lying completely still and quiet.

**Cuprum Met 6C to 30C -** First remedy to think of for heat exhaustion if the main symptom is *cramping or the person makes jerking motions of the muscles.* There may also be light-headedness, a rapid pulse and a cold sweat.

**Lycopodium 6C to 30C -** Heat exhaustion with gastric symptoms - flatulence or a heavy stomach immediately after eating and worse 4 - 8pm. They are generally better for uncovering and getting cooled down.

**Natrum Mur 6C to 30C -** Good for sunstroke with heat in the head and a red face, nausea and vomiting. A bursting headache or pain like 'tiny hammers' banging. There may be fiery zigzags before the eyes. Very thirsty and a marked desire or aversion to salty food.


BELOW FOR YOUR INTEREST IS THE OPINION OF A MASTER HOMOEOPATH. NOTE ACONITUM THE ONE THAT I AND A LOT OF OTHERS MISSED OUT, THAT'S WHY HE IS A MASTER. THIS IS REPEATED IN THE CATTLE SECTION.


## Heat Prostration for Cattle

**George MacLeod (McLeod) (1912 – 1995) MRCVS DVSM Veterinary FF. Hom**

### Sunstroke

Direct rays of the sun on the head may produce dilation of cerebral blood-vessels which in severe cases can cause paralysis. **Symptoms -** Excitement and restlessness are quickly evident and in the less acute case paralysis of certain muscles takes place, finally leading to failure of the respiratory centre.

### Homoeopathic Treatment

**Aconitum Napellus 12X.** This remedy given at once will help calm the animal and reduce excitement. Dose - one every half-hour for four doses.

**Beladonna 1M.** A most useful remedy for cerebral congestion. Generally there may be visible throbbing of surface vessels, with excitement and dilated pupils. Dose - One every half-hour for four doses. It should be alternated with Aconitum.

**Glonoine 30C.** One of the main remedies for exposure to sun. The animal exhibits signs of pain in the head, such as throwing the head against any convenient object or banging on the ground. Recumbency is usual with unsteadiness of movement if made to rise. This remedy will do much to reduce the tension in the cerebral blood vessels. Dose - one every hour for four doses.

# Heat Exhaustion

Accumulation of body heat may arise after exposure to a long spell of hot weather when the heat builds up in the body. It can be made worse by exercise. Factors which may influence this condition apart from heat are lack of proper oxygenation, fatigue, and insufficient intake of water, together with unnecessary handling, during prolonged hot weather. **Symptoms -** Rapid respirations are a constant sign along with depression and anorexia. The mouth is usually open and frothy mucus accumulates. A rapid pulse is present, while an extremely high temperature is constant. The conjunctivae become congested and motor reflexes are lost.

### Homoeopathic Treatment

**Glonoine 30C.** As Glonoine 30C for Sunstroke.

**Natrum Muriaticum 30C.** A useful remedy for stabilising the salt metabolism and preventing loss. Dose: one every three hours for four doses.

**Sulphur 30C.** This remedy is useful for reducing the effects of heat generally, enabling the animal to make a quicker recovery. Dose - one dose every two hours for four

doses. The administration of these remedies will help the action of cold water applications, which are always extremely valuable in reducing heat.

## Pigs and Heat Stress

Pigs are going to have a problem with climate change as they are unable to cool themselves with perspiration as humans can do, which makes them very susceptible to heat stress. Another problem is that they also get sunburnt, and should not be exposed to long periods of direct sunlight or extremes of temperature. Problems may begin at about 25 Celsius. Outdoor pigs survive the heat naturally by finding shady cool areas with a breeze and increasing water uptake along with lying on a cool surface. As the heat rises they would then start looking for places where they could make or find some where to make a mud bath, or head off to their local mud bath and have a roll in the mud to cool down with the mud also being their sun tan lotion. Pigs that are being fattened especially in summer can suffer heat stress from about 20 Celsius onwards, remember calories make heat. Signs of heat exhaustion in pigs can include open mouth breathing, panting and making more noise than usual, blotchy skin, stiffness, muscle tremors, and a reluctance to move. They will also reduce the amount of food they are consuming to slow the internal heat that is produced by digestion. When the animal starts panting very hard, that's when you are in trouble, especially if the heats going to last for a long time. A good start would be soaking a big towel with cold water and putting it on the pig's neck and back along with a long cool drink. Always check the young first as they are usually the ones that are affected first and the most, especially if mum stops producing milk, followed by the sows as they have a higher death rate during heat stress. Continuous access to clean water is critical for pig health. The key clinical signs and symptoms include a high respiratory rate, distress and a rectal temperature of 43°C. Part of the problem with pigs is that they don't sweat and they have small lungs so panting may not give much relief.

## Symptoms of Heat Stress

Respiration increases and may lead to panting.
Lethargic when moving, slowed down.
Feed intake is slowed so as to reduce internal heat.
Reduced growth in feeder pigs and maybe the young.
Reduced milk production in lactating sows.
General loss in weight.
Diarrhoea.
Increased water consumption.
Increased urine output.
Muscle trembling and weakness.

## Transporting Pigs during Hot Days

Hots days are not good for transporting pigs especially when it gets over 25 Celsius. It is best to avoid transporting pigs on hot or humid days. If you have to move them ensure they are transported in a covered and well ventilated trailer to avoid sunburn and to have a cooling breeze. The hotter it gets the more you have to reduce the loading density for example above 25C reduce loading by 10 percent and the hotter it gets consider more so as to allow the pigs to lie on the floor and ensure they are having a good breeze pass through them. On arrival unloaded immediately and give access to cool clean water and shade.

## Cattle and Heat Stress

As some places are more affected by climate change then others along with the related water changes due to the changing weather patterns, there will be many changes in the breeds of cattle as their suitability in certain areas becomes questioned. A lot of the British breeds are not going to like the heat and no doubt there will be a lot of experimenting with crossbreeds now and into the near future. Cattle are more prone to heat stress than sheep and goats. Beef cattle with black hair suffer more from direct solar radiation than those with lighter hair, while those with pink skin are at risk of sunburn. Lactating cattle are more susceptible than dry cows because of the additional metabolic heat generated during lactation while high producing dairy cows are more affected by extreme heat than lower producing cows. Heavy cattle over 450kg are more susceptible than lighter ones to sun and heat stroke and no doubt all the overweight ones are.

### Symptoms of Heat Stress

Reduced feed intake or change in feeding.

Cattle stand rather than lie down.

Bunching up in shaded areas.

Bunching up around the water trough.

Rapid shallow breathing or open mouth breathing.

Respiration rate increase with the heat.

Panting at higher temperatures.

Increased saliva production.

Lack of coordination and trembling.

Heatwaves can cause rapid dehydration in calves.

Sick or stressed cattle do not like heatwaves.

In regards to heat, cattle and cows do not sweat effectively and rely on respiration to cool themselves. To add to the burden the fermentation process within the rumen creates additional heat which accumulates during the day and dissipates at night when it is cooler. This creates a problem during heatwaves, especially if they last a long time and even worse when the temperatures just keep on going up. Cattles core temperature peaks 2 hours after the peak temperature of the day and then it takes at least 6 hours for their heat load to dissipate. Heavy cattle have a harder time with heat stress due to increased fat deposition and will need more time for recovery. As respiration is used for cooling keep your eyes open for animal's with respiratory problems as they will fare worse and like the canary in the cage they should give you the first warnings of what may come if the temperatures do not drop. Water is the fastest and quickest way for cattle to reduce their core body temperature so you have to ensure that they are able to get it which creates more problems. As we know that the climate is only going to get worse it should now be a priority to add more water troughs and more shady cool areas for stock and allow them the time they need to get used to the changes.

## Heat Prostration for Cattle

**George MacLeod (McLeod) (1912 – 1995) MRCVS DVSM Veterinary FF. Hom**

## Sunstroke

Direct rays of the sun on the head may produce dilation of cerebral blood-vessels which in severe cases can cause paralysis. **Symptoms -** Excitement and restlessness are quickly evident and in the less acute case paralysis of certain muscles takes place, finally leading to failure of the respiratory centre.

## Homoeopathic Treatment

**Aconitum Napellus 12X.** This remedy given at once will help calm the animal and reduce excitement. Dose - one every half-hour for four doses.

**Beladonna 1M.** A most useful remedy for cerebral congestion. Generally there may be visible throbbing of surface vessels, with excitement and dilated pupils. Dose - One every half-hour for four doses. It should be alternated with Aconitum.

**Glonoine 30C.** One of the main remedies for exposure to sun. The animal exhibits signs of pain in the head, such as throwing the head against any convenient object or banging on the ground. Recumbency is usual with unsteadiness of movement if made to rise. This remedy will do much to reduce the tension in the cerebral blood vessels. Dose - one every hour for four doses.

## Heat Exhaustion

Accumulation of body heat may arise after exposure to a long spell of hot weather when the heat builds up in the body. It can be made worse by exercise. Factors which may influence this condition apart from heat are lack of proper oxygenation, fatigue, and insufficient intake of water, together with unnecessary handling, during prolonged hot weather. **Symptoms -** Rapid respirations are a constant sign along with depression and anorexia. The mouth is usually open and frothy mucus accumulates. A rapid pulse is present, while an extremely high temperature is constant. The conjunctivae become congested and motor reflexes are lost.

### Homoeopathic Treatment

**Glonoine 30C.** As Glonoine 30C for Sunstroke.

**Natrum Muriaticum 30C.** A useful remedy for stabilising the salt metabolism and preventing loss. Dose: one every three hours for four doses.

**Sulphur 30C.** This remedy is useful for reducing the effects of heat generally, enabling the animal to make a quicker recovery. Dose - one dose every two hours for four doses. The administration of these remedies will help the action of cold water applications, which are always extremely valuable in reducing heat.

## Horses and Heat Stress

The best example we can use for Heat Stress is the racing horse. Exercise results in the generation of heat, and in a horse race the horses can produce enough heat to increase the body temperature by one degree Celsius for every minute of the race. For your average non-working horse its problems in climate change could be high temperatures and humidity, lack of wind or air movement in housing along with heat, poor ventilation and dehydration, while outside there would be exposure to direct sunlight and heat with maybe hot dry winds and not much shade. A horse's natural response to heat is usually to increase their sweating along with the rate of breathing and to move more blood into the capillaries under the skin so as to cool it a bit before entering the main blood stream again, that is of course if it didn't have a cold drink of water first.

### Symptoms of Heat Stress

Excessive or profuse sweating.
No sweating. (Runout of spare water).
Skin that is dry and hot.
Reduced feed intake.
Rapid shallow breathing or panting.
Flared nostrils.
Unpredictable behaviour and gait.
Very high body temperature.
High respiratory rate.
High heart rate – over 50 beats per minute.
High rectal temperature over 39 degrees Celsius.

A simple test to determine if the horse is dehydrated is to pinch the horse's skin on the neck and see if it resumes its original position immediately, if it takes a while to resume its normal position then it's dehydrated. As usual it is the old and young that can get into difficulties fairly fast so always keep an eye on them when it gets too hot. The very young and foals have a very poor heat regulating ability and can overheat just by standing in the sun so great care is needed for them especially if mum isn't all that bright. It is very worthwhile to have handy a large salt and electrolyte formula that you could use in emergencies, which should be easily found at any good horse shop. Horses that are overweight and not used regularly, along with not being used to hard work are some of the main victims of heat stroke. Horses with difficulty in breathing and looking stressed that develop diarrhoea or signs of colic, or stop sweating are in need of help. Take the horse to a cool and shady area and hose down the horse gently, if you fear the water is to cold sponge the horse down or do a mixture of both. As the horse settles direct the hose to the insides of the legs, head and neck areas following the areas where there are large blood vessels so as to help cool the blood, which in turn will help cool the body internally. Don't forget the wet towel trick especially for the young. Excess water must be scraped off afterwards unless there is a good breeze, as water in the coat on a hot, humid, still day will act as an insulator and it will quickly warm up again. You can use fans to cool and help evaporate the water which will increase the cooling. Offer a bit of water along with water dosed with electrolytes and let them choose which they want but slow them down if they get to greedy. Sometimes it can take an hour or more to get the temperature back to normal. Allow the horse to recover for about 10 days keeping a good eye on them. Restrict exercising your horse to the early morning and the cool of the evening when it is the coolest. If they liked and chose the Electrolytes before you can also add it to their feed regime for a few days to replace essential salts lost through sweating.

## Sheep and Heat Stress

Heat stress in sheep is a significant concern, more so in climate change where weather becomes unpredictable, unreliable and extremes become normal. Here the cold breeds will be affected the most as they tend to have shorter bodies and legs, short thick ears and denser fleeces, so these will have a very real risk of fatalities if signs are not recognised early and steps taken to reduce the risks. High temperatures will also affect feed intake, growth rates, fertility, conception rates and are often accompanied by high humidity which makes the situation worse. The hotter the summers get the more the fodder will be affected and to make it worse the rain may change its normal patterns and what may have been good pastures will turn not so good, maybe now is a good time for a rethink and a change in plans. As you know, plenty of fresh cool water is needed to keep sheep healthy and heat stress free, so now is the time to increase the number of troughs and shade so you are prepared for the worst, and save yourself from the problem of all the troughs being over crowed and causing problems. On average sheep will drink one to two gallons (3.7 litres to 7.4) of water a day, with lactating females needing more. Young animals need to drink more often as they have a faster metabolism but only a small tummy.

### Symptoms of Heat Stress

Shade seeking.

Crowding at water troughs.

Bunching to seek shade from other sheep.

1/. Open mouth breathing or panting.

2/. Head extended, tongue protruding, profuse salivation.

1 is the beginning, 2 is really bad.

Increased Respiration.
Increased Respiration with deep flank movements.
Wetting head in a water trough.
Weakness or inability to stand.
Rectal temperature above 41°C. (urgent)
Front legs held in a wide stance.

In extreme heat sheep will decrease their grazing time and spend more time in the shade, especially during the heat of the day, and will graze mostly in the evening and early morning hours. If you find heat-stressed animals move them to a cool, shaded area with good air circulation and for those that are in serious trouble with their head extended and tongue protruding it's time to start to lower body temperature. Sheep should be cooled by applying rubbing alcohol to the area between their rear legs as this area is not covered with wool and has a lot of vascular activity which means we will be cooling not only the skin but the blood as well, as it travels back to the heart. Don't accidently set the poor thing on fire by smoking or having it next to an electric fence. For sheep we do not wet the wool areas as this will actually make matters worse as air will not be able to pass through the fleece. With a hose carefully wet the underside and legs avoiding wool areas along with trying to get a breeze flowing in the same area. Work slowly but surely as you do not want to give a stressed animal the shock of a rapid change as that may be the end especially for the old and young. Other cooling treatments include ice applications and cool water enemas, but only do those for the first time with a vet who can show you how to do it properly and what to do if something goes wrong. Always offer heat-stressed sheep ample water and encourage them to drink small amounts and observe how they are handling it. If you have a water misting bottle it makes it easier to cool the legs and belly and any other place where there is no wool.

# Goats and Heat Stress

Goats are similar to sheep in heat stress especially the Angora Goats which like sheep have fleece and the problems that go with it, but have an advantage by having horns which can act like a cooling radiator in a car due to the amount of blood supply flowing through the horns. A cold pack wrapped around the horns may help with cooling but not a frozen one as we don't want give them a brain freeze. Other than the Angora, most goats handle the heat far better and a lot of them are breed for the heat such as the Anglo - Nubians who I helped farm in the tropics with their long floppy ears which help in cooling and long legs which keep them high from the grounds radiating heat. Lactating goats require more water in order to produce milk. As usual the very young and the very old goat will be less heat-tolerant, while the darker coloured goats attract more of the sun's heat and can overheat faster than a white goat. Sunburn can be a problem with light-skinned and coloured goats. Heat stress can lead to heat exhaustion or heat stroke. Providing shade and plenty of fresh water help most goat varieties avoid heat stress.

## Symptoms of Heat Stress

Shade seeking.

Crowding at water troughs.

Bunching to seek shade.

Open mouth breathing or panting.

The goats become lethargic.

Increased Respiration Rate.

Weakness or inability to stand.

Rectal temperature above 40°C. (urgent)

Similar to Sheep, Goats pant a lot when the weather is hot. If a goat can't stop panting, stops eating and drinking, and can't get up, it is most likely suffering from heat stress. Rectal temperatures over 40 degrees Celsius are a serious threat and cooling will need to be done along with shade, water and a cool area to recover. Non wool goats can be cooled down using water misting bottles or a fine mist hose especially on long floppy ears (be careful not to get water in the ears) and the horns which can act as cooling radiators along with spraying the rest of the body. If the air is not moving then bring out a few fans. Give the Goat access to cool clean water, small amounts regularly. The main method of transferring heat from a goat varies based upon the air temperature and **humidity,** which is the main killer in the equation. Evaporation will remove heat from the goat but it is critical that the humidity not be very high. Evaporation rates are increased when air passing above the coat has a lower humidity.

## Dogs and Working Dogs Heat Stress

Dogs don't sweat as humans do instead they release heat by panting and sweating through their paw pads and nose. If they cannot cool themselves their temperature begins to rise. Be aware of how hard your dog is working in the heat, especially when there is High Humidity. If the heat and humidity are high save the work for another day if you can, and always plan your work with the help of the weather forecast. If they must work, it should only be during the cool times of the day, and they must have regular breaks with access to water and shade. Carry water with you if possible and offer small amounts often. Stop work for a dog suspected of suffering from heat stress and check them out and offer water, if you are still worried put them in a water trough and cover their back with water and see how they react. If you are still not happy put them in the shade with a cool breeze if you can.

## Symptoms of Heat Stress

Heat stress – Increased thirst and panting

Dry nose (caused by dehydration)

Heat Exhaustion - Heavy Panting and Weakness

Heat Stroke – Drooling, Dizziness, Collapse.

Increased heart rate and breathing

May be vomiting and diarrhoea.

Muscle tremors and seizures.

Collapse.

Ensure your working dogs have access to shade and a source of clear fresh water at all times when they are kennelled or resting. Ice cubes in a dog's water bowl will help to keep water cool. Do not leave dogs tied up on the back of a ute in the sun and on days over 28C dogs must have a layer of insulating material between them and the metal tray. Always park in the shade and provide water and breeze if you can. Do not leave dogs locked in parked cars. Begin treatment for Heatstroke by moving the dog to a cool shaded area, hopefully with a breeze and begin cooling your dog by wetting down their body with a hose or bucket, but avoid the face. I used to start at the back using my hand to push the fur upward and a low pressure hose following and then do the sides. If there is no breeze then get a fan out to make one as we need the evaporation of the water to do the cooling. Keep doing this for a while and they will generally let you know when feeling better. For pets leave them at home during heatwaves as much as possible with plenty of water and shade and do not force the animal to exercise in hot, humid weather. Exercise pets in the cool of the early morning or evening so as to prevent foot burns from the tar on the roads and hot concrete. Because a dog is much closer to the ground hot asphalt and concrete can heat up quickly, and its paws can sustain burns or injuries. Dogs can get sunburned so protect hairless and light-coated dogs with sunscreen when they will be outside in the sun for an extended period of time. Put sunscreen or zinc on exposed areas of pink skin. Animals with long coats can be clipped to increase comfort in hot weather.

## Cats and Heat Stress

Heat exhaustion is the prelude to heatstroke, so you have to move fast before the condition deteriorates. Signs to look out for in Cats are restlessness and restless behaviour as they try to find a cool place, which is usually under the house lying on the cool soil and if they are lucky a nice breeze. Other signs are panting, excessive grooming, drooling, pacing up and down and sweaty paws which are all an effort to cool down. Heatstroke occurs in Cats at about 40 degrees Celsius

### Symptoms of Heat Stress

Panting or trouble breathing.
Panting increases.
Drooling, restlessness.
Diarrhoea.
Vomiting.
Staggering, Lethargy.
Muscle tremors, Seizures.
Increased Heart rate.
Disorientation.
Red flushed tongue or gums.
Little to no urine, Coma.

Cats that are at high risk of heat stroke are the old and young, those with a health problem, the fat cat and the flat faced breeds such as Persian or Burmese. Cats with long thick coats need to be trimmed before the heat of summer begins. Prevention is the best way to go especially if you know a heatwave is coming, find the coolest area in the house and set the cat up there with plenty of cool water. That should hopefully save them from burning their feet on hot concrete or tar or dehydrating in the hot breeze. Also on the worst hot days consider giving them wet cat food but in smaller amounts spread out during the day as this would take a lot of workload off the digestive system and keep up the hydration. Our old cat that was fairly bright always went under the house in hot weather and cooled herself on the nice cool soil. If you think your cat is suffering from heat stress take them inside to a cool room and have a feel of the floor temperature to see if it is cool. In severe cases where you know the cat is in trouble start with a temperature check which is done rectally with the normal temperature being just slightly over 38 degrees Celsius to 39.2. Temperatures over and above 40 degrees Celsius are a cause of alarm. Provide cool water and encourage them to drink, but not too much at a time. If the cat has had a drink but still looks bad then we have to cool them manually. Find a water bottle that can be used as a mister for spraying and gently and slowly spray the tummy and chest and get a fan set on low speed breezing into the tummy and chest area. If they are not complaining but seem to need more help you can get 2 hand towels and soak them in water and ring them out but not too much, then scruff the towels up and put the first one between the front paws and then point the fan at it but not too close and see what happens. What we are doing is using the evaporation to cool down the cat. If the cat is happy do the same with the rear legs and aim the fan at the middle of the cat. Adding a small amount of rubbing alcohol to the water can also help speed up the evaporation and cooling effect. Check the temperature every 10 minutes so you know what is happening.

# Poultry Heat Stress - Chickens

Here we will only deal with chickens as they are the most common small acreage and home reared poultry and are similar to turkeys in heat stress. Ducks and Geese will just take over the swimming pool in a heat wave and probably be happy in a bath tub under a shady tree. Chickens that are too hot will pant and spread their wings to release body heat. Panting releases water into the air which evaporates and helps to cool the chicken, but you can only do that for so long as eventually it will cause dehydration and a pH imbalance. High humidity decreases heat loss from the lungs which makes the birds more prone to heat stress. When the temperature starts to get to hot for chickens they naturally lose heat through their comb, wattles and other areas not covered by feathers and no doubt by a long cool drink. Poultry should not be wet down unless there is a breeze to aid the cooling process and increase air movement around them. This can be done with fans, ventilation, or wind movement. Warm water is less effective for cooling chickens and will cause fungi, mould, bacteria, and other microbes to grow in water which create other problems. You can also add electrolyte solutions to the drinking water in heat waves so as to help prolong the time till dehydration becomes a problem but only do this for no more than 3 days.

## Symptoms of Heat Stress

Panting.

Spreading Wings.

Increased thirst.

Lethargy – slowed down.

Decrease in egg laying.


Chickens do not have sweat glands so one of the main ways they try to cool down is by spreading their wings especially when there is a breeze around. If you see them doing this then it's time to get the fan out. Heat stress can cause a decrease in eggs as mentioned before but also dehydration which decreases the water in the egg and electrolytes in the body. Layers can also become calcium deficient which will cause the egg shells to become thinner and weaker. Chickens in heat can also lose weight and become susceptible to other diseases. A good rule of thumb is that when temperatures rise between 24 to 27 degrees C, it is time to check and begin cooling off your chickens. If temperatures are closer to 37 degrees or beyond, it can be dangerous. Always plan for the worst and hope for the best. During a heat wave feed chickens during the early morning or evening, the coolest parts of the day. Remember calories are a measure of heat, food actually makes you hotter. Keeping the coop cool is an excellent way to make sure your flock stays comfortable during hot weather. Regularly clean out litter as a build-up of litter that has started to decay produces heat, so by removing litter you lower the moisture in the coop, which reduces the relative humidity. Make sure your coop has grass around it and not bare dirt as grass absorbs heat, while dirt reflects heat. Always place a coop where there is a breeze as this is the best way to lower heat and keep up the ventilation. Keeping the water where the breeze exits the coops can help in reducing the humidity inside the coops. Air flow removes hot air and humidity. If you cannot get sufficient natural airflow install fans.

## Making your Own Fire Trailer

Here we will go back to the beginning. I saw my first Fire Trailer in use in 2006 on a farm I was living on in South Australia 50Ks north of Adelaide City. As it was very hot there was a fire ban. The area around Adelaide is very rocky which makes it very annoying for the farmers. In the early 18th century convicts starting working on the problem by clearing the fields of rocks and using the rocks to fence the paddocks. It was a good idea at the time but in the future it created a problem for tractors using slashers to keep the grass down as the paddocks were littered with small rocks which cause big sparks when the blades hit them which in turn starts fires that can get out of control fast especially if the wind picks up which seems to happen every time you hit a rock. In times of fire danger when you had to use the slasher you would hook up the fire trailer and park it in the middle of the paddock that you were slashing. The fire trailer was mostly made up of bits and pieces found around the farm and put together. The main bed for the equipment was an old 4x6 foot common trailer which had been strengthened on the floor so as to support the 1000 litre IBC tank and light chains each side with large fence strainers to tension the tank to the trailer. The wheels had 4wd tyres that were wider and stronger along with all the wheel bearings being renewed. This trailer had the petrol engine water pump at the front, mounted on the A frame of the trailer with the pump facing the trailer and the pump motor facing the vehicle. The main hose attached to the pump was the red standard fire hose that you would usually see on the walls of government buildings looking like a red circle on the wall with the black thin hose (Red Fire Hose Reel) which you can usually get very cheaply at the local auctions. Some people like the pump and hose at the front of the trailer while other like it at the back of the trailer. The 1000 litre IBC tank is 4 x 4 feet so on a 4 x 6 Trailer you have 2 feet at the back to mount the pump and the hose wheel. Make the mounting for the hose reel very strong so someone standing on the back can support themselves and use a hose at the same time as this is how they commonly put out the reoccurring spot fires with the driver heading to the fires and the person at the back putting them out. The design for your fire trailer is only limited by your imagination and must be set up by you for your own conditions and needs. You could do this as a joint project with your neighbours or other farmers in the area which could save you a lot of money with an example being buying your pump and other equipment in bulk for a discount which has another advantage of many people using the same equipment so they are familiar with it which is very helpful in emergencies. If you have a group networking together you could have a base station that could invest in a few drones that will give you the advantage of where the fires are in your area or when to run away. It's up to your imagination or for some just survival as this has been well and truly proved now and has saved many life's in Australia especially in the hills and ranges where the roads are easily blocked and the only ones that can save you are you and your neighbours. Don't forget fire trailers can also be used for lots of other purposes such as filling up long distance water troughs, mobile cleaning units, mobile cooling units for heat stressed animals or whatever your imagination come up with. We will end by showing you a cheap and basic modern unit designed solely for firefighting.

## BASIC - Pull Start - Fire Fighter 1000L Trailer A$2,241.00

Locally made Australian Galvanised Chassis

1350Kg Axles, Running Gear

Pull start 6.5hp generic engine (Remanufactured)

Up to 60m head (pumping vertically up)

Up to 8m suction (sucking vertically up)

Up to 200 Liters Per Minute

Reconditioned Firex Red Fire Hose Reel

36 Meter 19mm hose with brass twist nozzle

B-Grade Reconditioned IBC 1000 L Tank

Reconditioned Rims and Tyres

Economy clamp on Jockey Wheel

Mudguards

Fittings
https://egritech.square.site